Workbook to Accompany

UNDERSTANDING ANATOMY & PHYSIOLOGY

A Visual, Auditory, Interactive Approach

2nd edition

Workbook to Accompany

UNDERSTANDING ANATOMY & PHYSIOLOGY

A Visual, Auditory, Interactive Approach

2nd Edition

Gale Sloan Thompson, RN

F.A. Davis Company • Philadelphia

F. A. Davis Company
1915 Arch Street
Philadelphia, PA 19103
www.fadavis.com

Printed in the United States of America

Last digit indicates print number: 10 9 8 7 6 5 4 3 2 1

Publisher, Nursing: Lisa B. Houck
Director of Content Strategy: Darlene D. Pedersen
Content Project Manager II: Victoria White
Design and Illustration Manager: Carolyn O'Brien

As new scientific information becomes available through basic and clinical research, recommended treatments and drug therapies undergo changes. The author(s) and publisher have done everything possible to make this book accurate, up to date, and in accord with accepted standards at the time of publication. The author(s), editors, and publisher are not responsible for errors or omissions or for consequences from application of the book, and make no warranty, expressed or implied, in regard to the contents of the book. Any practice described in this book should be applied by the reader in accordance with professional standards of care used in regard to the unique circumstances that may apply in each situation. The reader is advised always to check product information (package inserts) for changes and new information regarding dose and contraindications before administering any drug. Caution is especially urged when using new or infrequently ordered drugs.

REVIEWERS

Tetteh Abbeyquaye, PhD
Assistant Professor
Quinsigamond Community College
Worcester, MA

Janice Ankenmann, RN, MSN, CCRN,
 FNP-C
Professor
Napa Valley College
Napa, CA

Dan Bickerton, MS
Instructor
Ogeechee Technical College
Statesboro, GA

Anne L. Brown, RN, BSN
Nursing Instructor
Broome-Tioga BOCES
Binghamton, NY

Susan E. Brown, MS, RN
Faculty
Riverside School of Health Careers
Newport News, VA

Henry Steven Carter, MS,
 CRC, CVE
*Coordinator of Continuing
 and Workforce Education/
 Instructor*
El Centro College
Dallas, TX

Thea L. Clark, RN, BS, MS
Coordinator Practical Nursing
Tulsa Technology Center
Tulsa, OK

Ginny Cohrs, RN, BSN
Nursing Faculty
Alexandria Technical College
Alexandria, MN

Tamera Crosswhite, RN, MSN
Nursing Instructor
Great Plains Technology Center
Frederick, OK

Fleurdeliza Cuyco, BS, MD
Dean of Education
Preferred College of Nursing, Los Angeles
Los Angeles, CA

Judith L. Davis, RN, MSN, FNP
Practical Nursing Instructor
Delta-Montrose Technical College
Delta, CO

Carita Dickson, RN
LVN Instructor
San Bernardino Adult School LVN
 Program
San Bernardino, CA

Teddy Dupre, MSN
Instructor
Capital Area Technical College
Baton Rouge, LA

Hisham S. Elbatarny, MB BCh,
 MSc, MD
Professor
St. Lawrence College—Queen's
 University
Kingston, Ontario

Alexander Evangelista
Adjunct Faculty
The Community College of Baltimore
 County
Baltimore, MD

John Fakunding, PhD
Adjunct Instructor
University of South Carolina, Beaufort
Beaufort, SC

Kelly Fleming, RN, BN, MSN
Practical Nurse Facilitator
Columbia College
Calgary, Alberta

Ruby Fogg, MA
Professor
Manchester Community College
Manchester, NH

Cheryl S. Fontenot, RN
Professor
Acadiana Technical College
Abbeville, LA

Shena Borders Gazaway, RN,
 BSN, MSN
Lead Nursing/Allied Health Instructor
Lanier Technical College
Commerce, GA

Daniel G. Graetzer, PhD
Professor
Northwest University
Kirkland, WA

Dianne Hacker, RN, MSN
Nursing Instructor
Capital Area School of Practical
 Nursing
Springfield, IL

Leslie K. Hughes, RN, BSN
Practical Nursing Instructor
Indian Capital Technology Center
Tahlequah, OK

Constance Lieseke, CMA (AAMA),
 MLT, PBT (ASCP)
*Medical Assisting Faculty Program
 Coordinator*
Olympic College
Bremerton, WA

Julie S. Little, MSN
Associate Professor
Virginia Highlands Community
College
Abingdon, VA

C. Kay Lucas, MEd, BS, AS
Nurse Educator
Commonwealth of Virginia
Department of Health
Professions
Henrico, VA

Barbara Marchelletta, CMA (AAMA),
CPC, CPT
Program Director, Allied Health
Beal College
Bangor, ME

Nikki A. Marhefka, EdM, MT (ASCP),
CMA (AAMA)
*Medical Assisting Program
Director*
Central Penn College
Summerdale, PA

Jean L. Mosley, CMA (AAMA),
AAS, BS
Program Director/Instructor
Surry Community College
Dobson, NC

Elaine M. Rissel Muscarella,
RN, BSN
LPN Instructor
Jamestown, NY

Brigitte Niedzwiecki, RN, MSN
*Medical Assistant Program Director
and Instructor*
Chippewa Valley Technical College
Eau Claire, WI

Jill M. Pawluk, RN, MSN
Nursing Instructor
The School of Nursing at Cuyahoga
Valley Career Center
Brecksville, OH

Kathleen Hope Rash, MSN, RN
*Curriculum & Instructional Resource
Coordinator*
Riverside Schools of Nursing
Newport News, VA

Amy Fenech Sandy, MS, MS
Dean, School of Sciences
Columbus Technical College
Columbus, GA

Marianne Servis, RN, MSN
Nurse Educator/Clinical Coordinator
Career Training Solutions
Fredericksburg, VA

Glynda Renee Sherrill, RN, MS
Practical Nursing Instructor
Indian Capital Technology Center
Tahlequah, OK

Cathy Soto, PhD, MBA, CMA
El Paso Community College
El Paso, TX

Joanne St. John, CMA
*Adjunct Instructor—Health
Science*
Indian River State College
Fort Pierce, FL

Diana A. Sunday, RN, BSN,
MSN/ED
*Nurse Educator—Practical Nursing
Program*
York County School of Technology
York, PA

Joyce B. Thomas, CMA (AAMA)
Instructor
Central Carolina Community
College
Pittsboro, NC

Marianne Van Deursen, MS Ed, CMA
(AAMA)
*Medical Assisting Program
Director/Instructor*
Warren County Community College
Washington, NJ

Monna L. Walters, MSN, RN
*Director of Vocational Nursing
Program*
Lassen Community College
Susanville, CA

Amy Weaver, MSN, RN, ACNS-BC
Instructor
Youngstown State University
Youngstown, OH

CONTENTS

INTRODUCTION

Most of us have one predominant learning style. Visual learners learn best when they can see a figure or an image; auditory learners prefer verbal explanations; kinesthetic learners need to incorporate movement into their learning time. Regardless, *everyone* can facilitate learning by employing a variety of techniques when studying, no matter their particular learning style.

Unlike any other study guide, the *Understanding Anatomy & Physiology* study guide is packed with unique activities involving drawing, coloring, and highlighting in addition to more traditional activities such as fill-in-the-blank and crossword puzzles. The drawing, coloring, highlighting, and writing activities give kinesthetic learners a chance to move, something they long to do when learning. Even if you're not primarily a kinesthetic learner, using your muscles will break up the monotony of studying and, by stimulating different parts of your brain, improve your learning experience. What's more, the colorful results of your drawing, coloring, and highlighting will provide quick, visual cues regarding important topics when you review.

To make the most of this study guide, you'll need at least 10 different colored pencils. Colored pencils will allow you to color various shades of each color, making them a better choice than colored pens. You'll also need an assortment of colorful highlighters, such as yellow, green, blue, and pink.

The following list summarizes the activities you'll find in this study guide:

- **Conceptualize in Color:** This activity involves coloring anatomical structures different colors. Kinesthetic learners will benefit from the movement associated with coloring as they focus on the various features of the human body, whereas visual learners will appreciate the visual aspect of coloring. Auditory learners can enhance their learning experience by saying the names of various structures out loud as they color. And, because coloring forces you to slow down and focus on one structure at a time, all learners will benefit.

- **Drawing Conclusions:** Combining drawing or coloring with some other activity, such as fill-in-the-blank sentences, "Drawing Conclusions" will hone your reasoning skills while allowing you to link written words

to something visual. The physical activity of drawing improves learning that much more.

- **Just the Highlights:** In this activity, you'll place sentences describing various structures, physiological processes, or disorders into separate groups by highlighting sentences in distinct colors. For example, in Chapter 5, *Integumentary System*, a "Just the Highlights" activity contains sentences describing features of first-, second-, and third-degree burns. You'll be asked to highlight sentences pertaining to first-degree burns in yellow, second-degree burns in orange, and third-degree burns in pink. Once complete, each group will be visually apparent, making reviewing easy.

- **Illuminate the Truth:** A variation of fill-in-the blank, you'll use a highlighter to identify the correct word or phrase that completes each sentence.

- **Fill in the Gaps:** In this fill-in-the-blank activity, you will write the correct word or phrase to complete each sentence. A Word Bank is provided.

- **Sequence of Events:** This activity will challenge you to place statements about a physiological process—such as the formation of cerebrospinal fluid—in proper sequence by inserting numbers in the blank line before each sentence.

- **Make a Connection:** This two-part activity involves first unscrambling words to reveal the names of certain structures or processes. Once identified, you'll draw a line from the word to a statement or description, linking the two together. For example, in Chapter 10, *Nervous System*, you'll unscramble words to discover the names of nervous system cells. You'll then draw lines to link the name of a cell to sentences describing characteristics of that type of cell.

- **List for Learning:** This activity will test your recall by asking you to make a list of certain things, such as the five functions of skin.

- **Puzzle It Out:** This traditional crossword puzzle is a fun way to test your knowledge of key terms related to anatomy and physiology.

- **Describe the Process:** Using figures as visual cues, you'll test your recall of physiological processes by describing the steps in a particular process, such as that of endochondral ossification. Successfully completing this activity will assure you that you have committed the process to memory.

Each activity in this book focuses on a specific topic. That way, if you are struggling in a particular area, you can choose the activities relating to that topic. After completing all the exercises for a chapter, consult the answer guide in the back of the book to check your answers.

Mastering the topic of anatomy and physiology requires study and repetition. There is no other way to construct the foundation of knowledge upon which you'll build your future career in health care. The unique activities in the *Understanding Anatomy & Physiology* study guide will aid you toward that end: They will break up the monotony of studying as you use color and movement to help you commit key facts to memory.

1 ORIENTATION TO THE HUMAN BODY

As you begin to study anatomy and physiology, you first need to understand how the body is organized. What's more, you need to learn the terms used to describe the various regions of the body. Doing the activities in this chapter will help.

List for Learning: Organization of the Body

The various elements of the human body are organized in a hierarchy ranging from the very simple to the very complex. Use the spaces below to list the major structures in this hierarchy, beginning with the atom and ending with the human organism.

1. Atoms

2. _____

3. _____

4. _____

5. _____

6. _____

7. _____

8. A human organism

Types of Tissue

Unscramble the words below to discover the names of the four types of tissue found in the human body. Then draw a line to link each type of tissue with its particular characteristics.

1. LEAPILEHIT

— — — — — — — — — — —

2. VICECENTON

— — — — — — — — — — —

3. CLESUM

— — — — — —

4. ENREV

— — — — —

A. Contracts to produce movement

B. Examples include the brain and nerves

C. Covers or lines body surfaces

D. Generates and transmits impulses to regulate body function

E. Connects and supports parts of the body; may also transport and store materials

F. Examples include the outer layer of the skin, the walls of capillaries, and kidney tubules

G. Examples include bone, cartilage, and adipose tissue

H. Examples include skeletal muscles and the heart

Use the figure above to complete the following instructions.

A. Draw a midline incision on the patient's abdomen, superior to the navel.

B. Draw a deep wound on the lateral portion of the right knee.

C. Draw a superficial wound on the medial right ankle.

D. Place a bandage on the proximal right arm.

E. Place an adhesive bandage on the left leg, distal to the knee.

F. Place a small bandage on the patient's abdomen, inferior to the navel.

Organ Systems

The human body consists of 11 organ systems, with each contributing to a particular function. Test your knowledge about these systems by completing the following crossword puzzle.

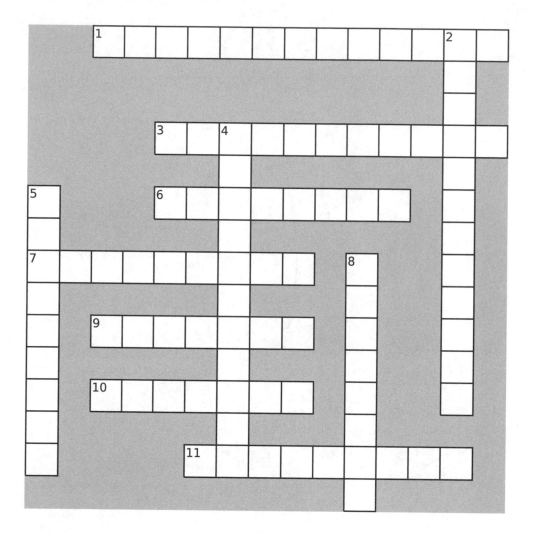

ACROSS

1. System consisting of skin, hair, and nails
3. System consisting of the heart, arteries, veins, and capillaries
6. System that participates in heat production
7. System involved in the breakdown and absorption of nutrients
9. System that helps regulate blood volume and pressure
10. System charged with the control, regulation, and coordination of other systems as well as sensation and memory
11. System that produces immune cells

DOWN

2. System consisting of the testes, vas deferens, prostate, seminal vesicles, and penis in males and the ovaries, fallopian tubes, uterus, vagina, and breasts in females
4. System consisting of the nose, pharynx, larynx, trachea, bronchi, and lungs
5. System involved in hormone production
8. System that plays a key role in blood formation

Body Planes

Test your knowledge of body planes by drawing the planes as instructed on the figure below. Then fill in the blanks to correctly describe each plane.

1. Draw a green square through the figure to illustrate a sagittal plane. Also called a _____

   plane, this plane divides the body into _____ and _____ sides.

2. Draw an orange square to divide the body into two halves using a transverse plane. Also called a

   _____ plane, this plane divides the body into _____ and

   _____ portions.

3. Draw a purple square through the body to illustrate a frontal plane. Also called a _____

   plane, this plane divides the body into _____ and _____ portions.

Various terms are used to describe different regions in the body. These terms are used extensively when performing clinical examinations and medical procedures. To help solidify your knowledge of the locations of these regions, color the figures below as described.

- Patellar area: Green
- Femoral area: Pink
- Pedal area: Yellow
- Gluteal area: Orange
- Palmar area: Orange
- Digital area: Green
- Scapular area: Pink
- Inguinal area: Green
- Axillary area: Blue
- Sacral area: Red
- Brachial area: Pink

- Deltoid area: Green
- Popliteal area: Green
- Sternal area: Red
- Pelvic area: Blue
- Pubic area: Yellow
- Antecubital area: Blue
- Buccal area: Yellow
- Occipital area: Red
- Lumbar area: Yellow
- Otic area: Blue
- Carpal area: Purple

The body's internal organs are contained in spaces called cavities. Color each cavity a color of your own choosing; then write the name of the cavity in the space provided.

Diaphragm

1. _____

2. _____

3. _____

4. _____

5. _____

6. _____

7. _____

8. _____

Because the abdominopelvic cavity is so large and because it contains numerous organs, it is divided into regions. Using the figure below, draw lines to divide this cavity into nine regions. Identify the names of the regions by coloring each region as described.

- Right hypochondriac region: Orange
- Left iliac region: Green
- Umbilical region: Yellow
- Right iliac region: Blue
- Left lumbar region: Brown
- Left hypochondriac region: Pink
- Right lumbar region: Purple
- Hypogastric region: Red
- Epigastric region: Gray

Next, identify the organs in each region by placing the correct letter in the proper square on the figure above. For example, if the small intestines, descending colon, and sigmoid colon are found in the right hypochondriac region, you would insert the letter A in that region on the figure.

A. Small intestines, descending colon, sigmoid colon

B. Small intestines, appendix, cecum, ascending colon

C. Pancreas, small intestines, transverse colon

D. Liver, gallbladder, right kidney

E. Stomach, liver (tip), left kidney, spleen

F. Stomach, liver, pancreas, right and left kidneys

G. Small intestines, descending colon, left kidney

H. Liver (tip), small intestines, ascending colon, right kidney

I. Small intestines, sigmoid colon, bladder

Review some key concepts from this chapter by highlighting the correct word or words in each of the following sentences.

1. The study of the structure of the body is called (physiology)(anatomy).

2. The smallest living units that make up the body's structure are called (organelles)(cells).

3. Structures of two or more tissue types that work together are called (organs)(organ systems).

4. Anatomical position is when the body is standing erect, arms at the sides, with palms facing (backward)(forward).

5. A disruption in one organ system usually has (no effect on) (consequences in) other systems.

Fill in the Gaps: **Homeostasis**

To maintain a stable environment, the body must constantly monitor conditions and make adjustments as conditions change. This process is called homeostatic regulation. Review this crucial process by filling in the blanks to complete each of the following sentences. Choose from the words listed in the Word Bank below. (Hint: Not all the words will be used.)

AMPLIFIES	**EQUILIBRIUM**	**POSITIVE**	**REVERSES**
CONTROL CENTER	**NEGATIVE**	**RECEPTOR**	**SUPPRESSES**
EFFECTOR	**OPPOSES**	**REINFORCES**	

1. Homeostasis is the state of dynamic _____ of the internal environment of the body.

2. To maintain homeostasis, a system must have three components: (1) a _____, which detects external changes that could influence the environment; (2) a _____, which receives and processes the information from the first component; and (3) a _____, which responds to signals from the second component by either opposing or enhancing the stimulus.

3. Negative feedback is when the effector _____ the stimulus and _____ the direction of change.

4. Positive feedback is when the effector _____ the stimulus and _____ the direction of change.

5. Most systems supporting homeostasis operate by _____ feedback.

2

CHEMISTRY OF LIFE

The human body is made of chemicals. What's more, life depends upon a precise balance between all those chemicals. So before you can understand how the body functions, you must have a firm grasp on how the chemicals in the body interact. The exercises in this chapter should help you do just that.

Illuminate the Truth: Basic Structures

Highlight the word or phrase that correctly completes each sentence.

1. An element's atomic number is determined by the (number of protons)(number of neutrons) in the nucleus.

2. An element's atomic weight is determined by adding the number of (protons, neutrons, and electrons)(protons and neutrons).

3. The number of electrons equals the number of (protons)(protons and neutrons added together).

4. Atoms are electrically (neutral)(positive).

5. The number of electron rings, or shells, (varies)(is the same) between atoms.

6. (All)(Some) isotopes of an element are unstable and emit radiation as they decay.

7. An element's unique chemical properties result from (the various combinations of protons, neutrons, and electrons)(the various types of protons, neutrons, and electrons making up the atoms of the element).

Chemistry Terms

Test your knowledge of general chemistry terms by completing the crossword puzzle below.

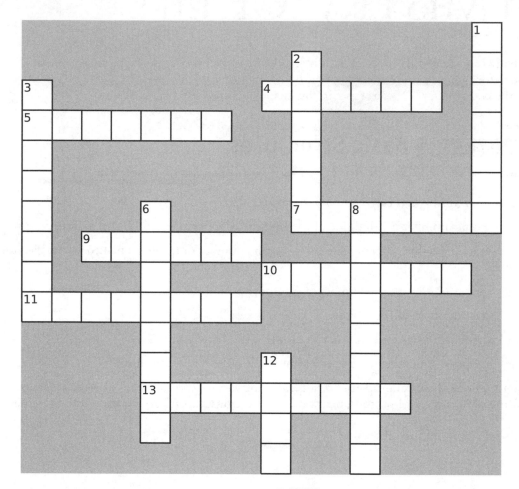

ACROSS

4. Anything that has mass and occupies space
5. An atom of an element that contains a different number of neutrons
7. Center of an atom
9. Element represented by the letter *O*
10. A pure substance that can't be broken down or decomposed into two or more substances
11. Particles in the center of an atom that carry a negative charge
13. Tiny particles that whirl around the center of an atom

DOWN

1. Particles in the center of an atom that carry a positive charge
2. Element represented by the letter *C*
3. One of the four elements that comprise the body: carbon, hydrogen, oxygen, and _____
6. Element represented by the letter *H*
8. Chemical combinations of two or more elements
12. Smallest part of an element

Drawing Conclusions: Chemical Bonds

First identify the key characteristics of ionic, covalent, and hydrogen bonds by filling in the blanks in the following sentences. Then, in the space provided, draw an example of each type of bond.

1. *Ionic Bonds*

Ionic bonds are formed when one atom (a) _____ an electron from its outer shell to

another atom. The electrical charge of the atom then changes from (b) _____ to either

(c) _____ or (d) _____.

Draw an example of an ionic bond between sodium and chlorine atoms in the space provided. An illustration of a sodium and chlorine atom has been provided to get you started.

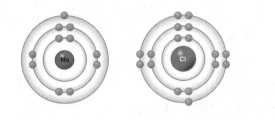

2. *Covalent Bonds*

In covalent bonds, two atoms (a) _____ one or more pairs of electrons. Covalent bonds are

(b) _____ than ionic bonds.

Draw an example of a double covalent bond between carbon and oxygen atoms to form CO_2. An illustration of a carbon and oxygen atom has been provided to get you started.

3. *Hydrogen Bonds*

A hydrogen bond is a weak (a) _____ between a slightly positive (b) _____ atom in

one molecule and a slightly negative (c) _____ or (d) _____ atom in another.

Using the illustration of a water molecule (shown here), draw an example of a hydrogen bond between two water molecules.

Unscramble the words on the left to reveal the three types of chemical reactions. Then draw lines to link each type with its particular characteristics.

1. HENSISSTY

_ _ _ _ _ _ _ _ _

2. OPTICDOMINOES

_ _ _ _ _ _ _ _ _ _ _ _ _

3. HANGEXEC

_ _ _ _ _ _ _ _

a. Involves the breakdown of a complex substance into two or more simpler substances

b. Requires energy input

c. Represented by the equation AB + CD →AC + BD

d. Occurs when two molecules exchange atoms or groups of atoms, forming two new compounds

e. Involves the combination of two or more substances to form a different, more complex substance

f. Represented by the equation AB →A + B

g. Releases energy

h. Represented by the equation A + B → AB

Puzzle It Out: Chemistry Concepts

Hone your knowledge of chemistry concepts by completing the following crossword puzzle.

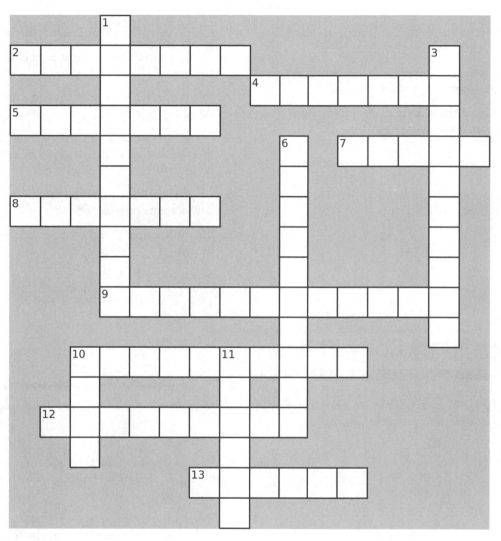

ACROSS

2. Particle composed of two or more atoms united by a chemical bond
4. The electrons in an atom's outer shell
5. Energy in motion
7. Type of molecule with an uneven distribution of electrons
8. Atoms having a positive charge
9. Compounds that ionize in water to create a solution capable of conducting electricity
10. Process whereby ionic bonds dissociate in water to create a solution of positively and negatively charged particles

12. Involves building larger and more complex chemical molecules, which requires energy input
13. The capacity to do work

DOWN

1. Reactions that can go in either direction under different circumstances
3. All the chemical reactions in the body
6. Involves breaking down complex compounds into simpler ones, releasing energy in the process
10. Electrically charged atoms
11. Atoms having a negative charge

Chapter 2 Chemistry of Life   *15*

Characteristics of Water

Unlike any other fluid, water has a number of characteristics that make it essential for life. Link the characteristics of water with its performance in the body by highlighting each of the following sentences as suggested.

- Highlight in pink the sentences describing water's action as a solvent.

- Highlight in yellow the sentences describing water's action as a lubricant.

- Highlight in blue the sentences describing water's ability to absorb and release heat.

1. Cells receive the chemicals they need to function.

2. The heart beats freely without encountering friction.

3. Joints operate smoothly, allowing the body to move.

4. The body can maintain a stable temperature despite changes in activity level or environmental temperature.

5. Large chemical compounds are broken down into components cells can use.

6. The lungs expand and contract freely for effortless breathing.

7. Sweat cools the body.

Make a Connection: # Body Fluids

Unscramble the words on the left to discover two types of fluid. Then draw lines linking each fluid type to its characteristics as well as to examples of each.

1. DOCUMPON

 _ _ _ _ _ _ _ _

2. REMITUX

 _ _ _ _ _ _ _

a. Results when two or more mixtures blend together, with each retaining its own chemical properties

b. Results when two or more elements combine to make a new substance that has its own chemical properties

c. Substances involved can be separated

d. Example: Table salt

e. Example: Water

f. Example: Salt in scrambled eggs

g. Example: Lemonade

Types of Mixtures

Mixtures of substances in water can be solutions, colloids, or suspensions. Identify the characteristics of each by highlighting each of the following sentences as suggested.

- Highlight in yellow the sentences describing solutions.
- Highlight in orange the sentences describing colloids.
- Highlight in blue the sentences describing suspensions.

1. Usually consist of a mixture of protein and water
2. Contain large particles, causing them to be cloudy or opaque
3. May be gas, solid, or liquid
4. Can change from a liquid to a gel
5. Are clear, with no visible particles; particles don't separate when the mixture is allowed to stand
6. Have particles that separate if the solution is allowed to stand
7. Contain particles small enough to stay permanently mixed but large enough to make the mixture cloudy
8. Example in the body: Glucose in the blood
9. Example in the body: Blood cells in plasma
10. Example in the body: Albumin in blood plasma

The pH Scale

Fill in the blanks with the appropriate words to complete each sentence. Choose from the words listed in the Word Bank below.

ACID	ACCEPTORS	BASE	DONORS	HYDROXIDE (OH⁻)
ACIDIC	ALKALINE	BASIC	HYDROGEN (H⁺)	NEUTRAL

1. Solutions with a pH less than 7 are _____.

2. Solutions with a pH greater than 7 are _____ or _____.

3. When acidic solutions are dissolved in water, they release _____ ions.

4. Alkaline solutions release _____ ions when dissolved in water.

5. Acidic solutions are called proton _____.

6. Alkaline solutions are called proton _____.

7. The greater the concentration of hydrogen (H^+) ions, the stronger the _____.

8. The greater the concentration of hydroxide (OH^-) ions, the stronger the _____.

9. A solution containing equal numbers of H^+ and OH^- ions is known as a _____ solution.

Illuminate the Truth: Organic Compounds

Highlight the word or phrase that correctly completes each sentence.

1. The term *organic* is used to describe compounds (containing carbon)(without carbon).

2. (Proteins)(Carbohydrates) are the body's main energy source.

3. Monosaccharides, disaccharides, and polysaccharides are all types of (carbohydrates)(fats).

4. The primary form of sugar found in the body is (glycogen)(glucose).

5. The stored form of glucose is (galactose)(glycogen).

6. Triglycerides, the most abundant lipid in the body, (serve no known purpose and are a major contributor to heart disease)(function as a concentrated source of energy).

7. Saturated fatty acids (form a solid mass)(are liquid) at room temperature.

8. Cholesterol is the body's chief (steroid)(triglyceride).

9. (Proteins)(Fats) are the most abundant, and most important, organic compound in the body.

10. Nonessential amino acids are so named because they (are not necessary for normal body function)(can be manufactured by the body).

11. Proteins consist of (electrolytes)(amino acids) linked together by peptide bonds.

12. Unsaturated fatty acids are derived mostly from (animal)(plant) sources.

13. A protein's function is determined by (the number of amino acids it contains)(its shape).

List for Learning: Lipids

List five major roles that lipids fulfill in the body.

1. _____

2. _____

3. _____

4. _____

5. _____

Unscramble the words below to reveal the names of some of the body's proteins. Then draw a line linking each of the proteins to its function.

1. TEARINK

   — — — — — — —

2. BIASEDINTO

   — — — — — — — — — —

3. NILISNU

   — — — — — — —

4. NIMBLEGOHO

   — — — — — — — — — —

5. CLEANLOG

   — — — — — — — —

6. SNEZEMY

   — — — — — — —

a. Defend the body against bacteria

b. Carries oxygen in the blood

c. Strengthens nails, hair, and skin

d. Gives structure to bones, cartilage, and teeth

e. Serves as a chemical messenger to cells throughout the body

f. Act as catalysts for crucial chemical reactions

List for Learning: **Cholesterol**

List four key roles cholesterol fulfills in the body.

1. _____

2. _____

3. _____

4. _____

Glucose and Glycogen

Fill in the blanks in the following paragraph to clarify how the body uses its prime energy source. Choose from the words listed in the Word Bank below. (Hint: Some words are used multiple times.)

GLUCOSE	**GLYCOGEN**	**LIVER**	**MUSCLES**

When blood (1)_____ levels are high (such as after eating), the (2)_____

converts excess (3)_____ into (4)_____, which it then stores. When blood

(5)_____ levels drop (such as between meals), the (6)_____ converts

(7)_____ back into (8)_____ and releases it into the blood. This keeps blood

(9)_____ levels within normal limits and provides cells with a constant supply of energy. The

(10)_____ also store (11)_____ to meet its energy needs during physical exercise.

ATP

Cells use energy in the form of ATP. Test your understanding of how the body's cells obtain and then restore their supply of energy by describing the process in the spaces provided. Use the illustrations as a guide. To get you started, the first part of each sentence is provided for each illustration.

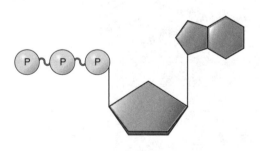

1. ATP consists of _____

_____ .

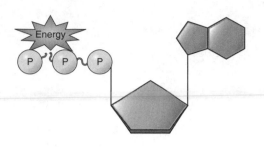

2. When one of the bonds is broken through a chemical reaction, _____ _____ .

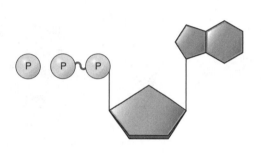

3. After the bond is broken, _____ _____ .

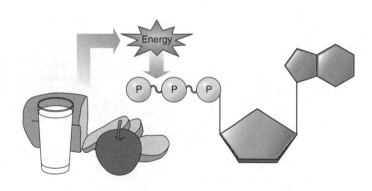

4. Meanwhile, the cell uses _____ _____ .

3
CELLS

Cells may be microscopic, but they are far from simple. In fact, each cell is packed with specialized structures that allow it to perform various tasks crucial to human life. Use this chapter to enhance your understanding of cellular structure and function. Doing so is the key to understanding the inner workings of the body, in both health and disease.

Conceptualize in Color: The Cell

Identify the various structures in a human cell by coloring the figure below. Use the suggested colors or choose colors of your own.

- Plasma membrane: Blue
- Nucleus and nuclear envelope: Purple
- Nucleolus: Dark blue

- Centriole: Green
- Mitochondria: Pink
- Golgi apparatus: Orange

- Smooth endoplasmic reticulum: Brown
- Rough endoplasmic reticulum: Tan

- Lysosomes: Red
- Ribosomes: Black
- Cytoplasm: Yellow

Plasma Membrane

Test your knowledge of the plasma membrane by filling in the blanks in the following sentences. Choose from the words listed in the Word Bank below. (Hint: Words may be used more than once; also, not all the words will be used.)

AWAY FROM	GLUCOSE	PHOSPHOLIPIDS	SELECTIVELY PERMEABLE
CHOLESTEROL	LOVING	POROUS	SUBSTANCES
FEARING	PASSAGE	PROTEIN(S)	TOWARD

1. Besides defining the boundaries of the cell, the plasma membrane regulates the _____ of _____ into and out of the cell.

2. The plasma membrane consists of _____, _____, and _____.

3. The heads of the phospholipids are water _____, causing them to face _____ the fluid in the cell's interior and exterior.

4. The tails of the phospholipids are water _____, causing them to face _____ the fluid in the cell's interior and exterior.

5. _____ molecules stiffen and strengthen the plasma membrane.

6. _____ are embedded in various spots in the membrane and fulfill a number of roles.

7. Because some substances can easily pass through the membrane, while others cannot, the plasma membrane is called _____ _____.

Proteins and the Plasma Membrane

Using the spaces provided, describe the three roles fulfilled by proteins in the plasma membrane.

1. _____

2. _____

3. _____

Cellular Structures

Complete the following crossword puzzle to enhance your learning of cellular structures and their functions.

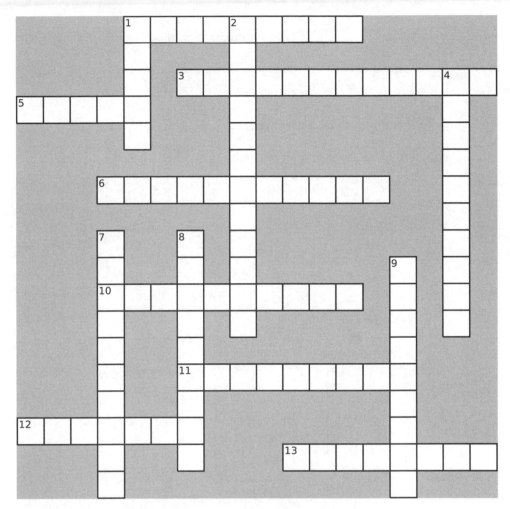

ACROSS

1. Thread-like structures composed of DNA and protein extending throughout the nucleus
3. Supporting framework of the cell
5. Apparatus that prepares and packages proteins for export to other parts of the body
6. Rod-like structures consisting of tightly coiled DNA
10. Bundles of microtubules that participate in cell division
11. Cellular garbage disposals
12. The cell's control center
13. Whip-like projection that helps move a cell

DOWN

1. Hair-like processes that propel substances along a cell's surface
2. The cell's powerhouses
4. Structures filling the cytoplasm that perform specific tasks in cellular metabolism
7. Folds of the cell membrane that greatly increase a cell's surface area
8. Gel-like substance that fills the space between the plasma membrane and nucleus
9. Cell's protein-producing structures

Diffusion

Fill in the blanks in the following sentences to demonstrate your knowledge of diffusion. Then use the accompanying figure to draw the process.

1. Diffusion is a _____ transport mechanism, meaning that it doesn't require energy.

2. Diffusion involves the movement of particles from an area of _____ concentration to an area of _____ concentration.

3. The point at which no further diffusion occurs is called _____.

4. A difference in concentration of a substance from one point to another is called a _____ _____.

Dye tablet

Time

Drawing Conclusions: Osmosis

Fill in the blanks in the following sentences to demonstrate your knowledge of osmosis. Then draw the process of osmosis in the empty container shown here.

1. Osmosis involves the diffusion of _____ across a selectively permeable membrane from an area of _____ to _____ concentration.

2. In the body, osmosis occurs when a particular substance _____ cross the cell membrane.

3. This process helps make the concentration of solutes _____ on both sides of the plasma membrane.

4. As water diffuses by osmosis into a solution, the _____ of that solution increases.

5. Water pressure that develops in a solution as a result of osmosis is called _____

   _____.

5% Albumin   10% Albumin

Side A   Side B

Illuminate the Truth: Tonicity

Highlight the word or phrase that correctly completes each sentence.

1. Tonicity is the ability of a solution to affect the (fluid volume)(solute concentration) and pressure in a cell through osmosis.

2. An isotonic solution contains a concentration of solutes that is (greater than)(the same as) the concentration of solutes inside the cell.

3. A hypertonic solution contains a (higher)(lower) concentration of solutes compared with the fluid in the cell.

4. A hypotonic solution contains a (higher)(lower) concentration of solutes compared with the fluid in the cell.

5. When a blood cell is placed in an isotonic solution, fluid moves into the cell (faster than)(at the same rate as) it moves out of the cell.

6. When a red blood cell is placed in a hypertonic solution, it (swells)(shrivels).

7. When a red blood cell is placed in a hypotonic solution, it (swells)(shrivels).

8. If infused into the human body, distilled water acts as a (hypotonic)(hypertonic) solution.

9. If infused into the human body, a concentrated salt solution would act as a (hypotonic)(hypertonic) solution.

10. Normal saline is considered (a hypotonic)(an isotonic) intravenous solution.

Fill in the Gaps: Filtration and Facilitated Diffusion

Fill in the blanks to complete each sentence. Choose from the words listed in the Word Bank below. (Hint: Not all of the words will be used.)

CAPILLARIES	**CONCENTRATION**	**PRESSURE**
CHANNEL PROTEIN	**MITOCHONDRION**	**VEINS**

1. In filtration, water and dissolved particles move from an area of higher to lower _____.

2. Filtration is the method used by _____ to deliver water and nutrients to the body's tissues.

3. In facilitated diffusion, molecules move from an area of higher to lower _____.

4. In facilitated diffusion, a solute enters a _____ to pass through the plasma membrane.

Drawing Conclusions: Sodium-Potassium Pump

Identify the following structures by coloring them as described in the figures below:

- Channel proteins:
  Purple

- Sodium molecules:
  Orange

- Potassium molecules:
  Green

- Extracellular area:
  Blue

Insert arrows by the molecules to show the direction of flow. Then, using each illustration as a guide, describe the four steps in the sodium–potassium pump in the spaces provided.

A.

Extracellular

Intracellular

1. _____
_____
_____
_____
_____
_____
_____
_____
_____
_____

B.

ATP

2. _____
_____
_____
_____
_____
_____
_____
_____
_____

C.

3. _____
_____
_____
_____
_____
_____
_____
_____

D.

4. _____
_____
_____
_____
_____
_____
_____
_____

Vesicular Transport

Unscramble the following words to reveal terms associated with transport by vesicles. Then draw lines to link each term to its characteristics.

1. SCOOTEDYINS

_ _ _ _ _ _ _ _ _ _ _ _

2. ACHOOSPIGSTY

_ _ _ _ _ _ _ _ _ _ _ _

3. OPTICSNOISY

_ _ _ _ _ _ _ _ _ _ _

4. SOCIETYSOX

_ _ _ _ _ _ _ _ _ _

a. Occurs when vesicles release substances outside the cell

b. Occurs when the cell engulfs a solid particle and brings it into the cell

c. General type of vesicular transport that brings substances into the cell

d. Occurs when vacuoles bring droplets of extracellular fluid containing dissolved substances into the cell

e. An example is when mammary glands secrete breast milk

f. Method used by white blood cells

DNA

List the four nitrogenous bases found in DNA. Then draw circles around the names of two bases that pair together and a square around the names of the other two bases that pair together.

1. _____

2. _____

3. _____

4. _____

DNA

Highlight the correct word or phrase to complete each sentence.

1. DNA molecules (store all of a cell's genetic information)(contribute to energy production in the cell).

2. DNA forms a dense coil that resembles an *X* (at all times)(when the cell is preparing to divide).

3. The sugar in DNA is (ribonucleic acid)(deoxyribose).

4. The sequence of bases in DNA is (predetermined)(varied); it's this sequence of bases that (provides the genetic code)(allows DNA to replicate).

5. One of DNA's main functions is to provide information for building (lipids)(proteins).

List for Learning: **RNA**

List three ways RNA differs from DNA.

1. _____

2. _____

3. _____

Sequence of Events: **Transcription**

Following are the various steps in the transcription process. Place the steps in the proper sequence by inserting numbers in the spaces provided: Insert number 1 by the first step, number 2 by the second step, etc.

_____ **A.** The mRNA begins the process of translation.

_____ **B.** The nucleus receives a chemical message to make a new protein.

_____ **C.** The mRNA separates from the DNA molecule and moves through a nuclear pore and into the cytoplasm.

_____ **D.** An RNA enzyme assembles RNA nucleotides that would be complementary to the exposed bases.

_____ **E.** The segment of DNA with the relevant gene unwinds.

_____ **F.** RNA nucleotides attach to the exposed DNA and then bind to each other to form messenger RNA (mRNA).

Translation

1. After the mRNA enters the cytoplasm, it attaches to (the Golgi apparatus)(a ribosome), which begins the process of translating the protein.

2. The mRNA carries the code for each amino acid in a series of three bases, called a (codon)(chromosome).

3. Each tRNA consists of (one base)(three bases).

4. The tRNA deposits (three amino acids)(a single amino acid) at the complementary site.

5. The (ribosome/mRNA) uses enzymes to attach the chain of amino acids together with (cholesterol)(peptide) bonds.

Cell Cycle

Unscramble the following words to discover the names of the four phases of the cell cycle. Then use lines to link each phase to its particular characteristics.

1. NESTISSHY

   _ _ _ _ _ _ _ _ _

2. CODENS PAG

   _ _ _ _ _ _ _   _ _ _

3. TICOMIT

   _ _ _ _ _ _ _

4. RIFTS PAG

   _ _ _ _ _ _   _ _ _

a. The cell is busy performing the tasks it was created to do.

b. Cell division occurs.

c. The cell synthesizes enzymes necessary for division.

d. The cell accumulates materials necessary for DNA replication.

e. The cell makes an extra set of DNA.

Following are illustrations of four cells in various stages of mitosis. In the blank to the right of each cell, write the name of each phase and describe what is occurring.

A.

_____
_____
_____
_____
_____

B.

_____
_____
_____
_____
_____

C.

_____
_____
_____
_____
_____

D.

_____
_____
_____
_____
_____

4

TISSUES

All the trillions of cells of the body can be categorized as belonging to one of four distinct groups of tissue. Remember: Tissues are simply groups of similar cells that perform a common function. Complete the exercises in this chapter to strengthen your knowledge of the four categories of tissue: epithelial, connective, nervous, and muscular.

Drawing Conclusions: Epithelial Tissue (Single Layer)

Fill in the blanks to complete the following sentences about the different types of epithelial tissue having one layer. (Hint: Some blanks require more than one word.) Next, color and then label each of the sample epithelial drawings.

1. Epithelial tissue having only one layer is called _____.

2. _____ epithelium consists of a single layer of flat, scale-like cells.

3. _____ epithelium consists of a single layer of cube-like cells.

4. _____ epithelium consists of a single layer of irregularly shaped columnar cells; the different cell heights make the tissue appear to be stratified.

5. _____ epithelium consists of a single layer of columnar cells.

A. _____

B. _____

C. _____

D. _____

Stretch your knowledge of tissues by completing this crossword puzzle.

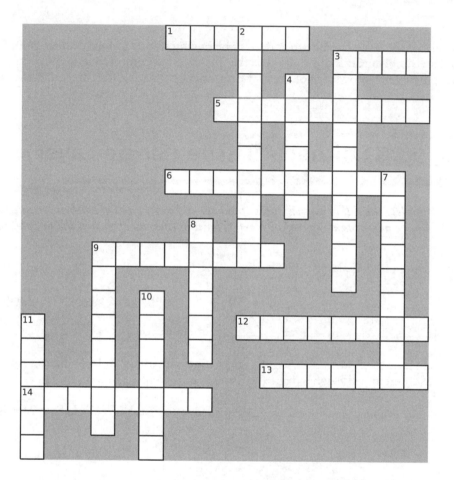

ACROSS

1. Dense connective tissue band or sheet that binds organs and muscles together

3. Type of cell that can differentiate into a number of different cells

5. Gland that secretes its product directly into the bloodstream

6. Tissue that lacks blood vessels and depends on underlying connective tissue for oxygen and nutrients

9. The body's most abundant protein

12. Gland that secretes its product into ducts

13. Tissue dominated by fat cells

14. Cell shape that is flat and plate-like

DOWN

2. The most widespread and most varied of all the tissues

3. Tissue that has multiple layers in which some cells don't touch the basement membrane

4. Modified cells containing secretory vesicles that produce large quantities of mucus

7. Cord-like tissues that attach bones to bones

8. Key component of connective tissue

9. Cell shape that is tall and cylindrical

10. Dense, cord-like tissues that attach muscles to bones

11. Groups of cells that perform a common function

Epithelial Function

In the following lists, link each type of epithelial tissue to its location in the body by highlighting each with the same color. For example, highlight "simple squamous epithelium" in blue; then highlight the body location where simple squamous epithelium is found in blue. Choose a different color for each type of epithelial tissue.

1. Simple squamous epithelium

2. Simple cuboidal epithelium

3. Simple columnar epithelium

4. Pseudostratified columnar epithelium

a. Lines the intestines

b. Lines the trachea, large bronchi, and nasal mucosa

c. Lines the alveoli

d. Lines the ducts and tubules of many organs, including the kidneys

Epithelial Tissue (Several Layers)

Color each of the following tissue samples. Beneath each figure, identify the tissue type and list at least one location where the tissue can be found.

1.

Tissue Type _____

Location in the Body _____

2.

Tissue Type _____

Location in the Body _____

Color and then label the following tissue samples. (**Hint:** Use your textbook if necessary to help you choose colors.)

A. _____

E. _____

B. _____

F. _____

C. _____

G. _____

D. _____

Differentiate between the traits of various tissues by highlighting the sentences different colors, as suggested:

- The sentences relating to epithelial tissues: Pink
- The sentences relating to connective tissue: Blue
- The sentences relating to muscle tissue: Orange
- The sentences relating to nervous tissue: Yellow

1. Glands are made of this tissue.

2. This tissue consists of elongated cells that contract in response to stimulation.

3. The cells of this tissue are embedded in an extracellular matrix.

4. This tissue contains no blood vessels and depends upon underlying connective tissue to supply its needs for oxygen and nutrients.

5. Types of this tissue include blood, bone, cartilage, and fat.

6. This tissue is found in the brain, spinal cord, and nerves.

7. This tissue forms the epidermis of the skin.

8. This tissue contains various types of fibers.

9. Tendons and ligaments consist of this type of tissue.

10. This type of tissue has a high degree of excitability and conductivity.

11. The key functions of this tissue involve protection, absorption, filtration, and secretion.

12. Three types of this tissue include skeletal, cardiac, and smooth.

13. This tissue serves to connect the body together and to support, bind, or protect organs.

Connective Tissue

Highlight the word or phrase that correctly completes each sentence.

1. (Collagenous)(Reticular) fibers occur in networks and support small structures, such as capillaries and nerves.

2. (Collagenous)(Elastic) fibers are the most abundant fibers in connective tissue.

3. Connective tissue is classified according to its (cell layers)(structural characteristics).

4. (Areolar)(Adipose) is a type of loose connective tissue found underneath almost all epithelia.

5. (Adipose)(Reticular) tissue forms the framework of the spleen, lymph nodes, and bone marrow.

6. (Cartilage)(Bone) is a type of dense connective tissue that has no blood supply, making healing slow or absent following an injury.

7. (Elastic cartilage)(Fibrocartilage) resists compression and absorbs shock, making it ideal to form the discs between the vertebrae.

8. The matrix of (bone)(cartilage) serves as a storage site for calcium.

9. Unlike other connective tissues, (bone)(blood) doesn't contain any fibers.

10. Most connective tissue has a (rich)(limited) blood supply.

Drawing Conclusions: **Tissue Repair**

Demonstrate your knowledge of tissue repair by coloring the illustration (which depicts the various stages in tissue repair) according to the following instructions. Then use the spaces below each figure to describe what's occurring in each step.

Use different colors as suggested to color the following figure:

- Wound: Dark red
- Scab: Brown
- Granulation tissue: Pink
- White blood cells: Purple
- New cells: Tan
- Scar tissue: White
- Fibroblasts: Orange

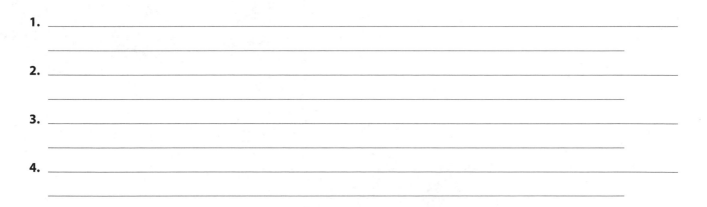

1. _____

_____

2. _____

_____

3. _____

_____

4. _____

_____

Unscramble the following words to reveal the names of the three types of epithelial membranes. Then draw lines to link each membrane with its characteristics.

1. CUMSOU

— — — — — —

2. SAUCEUNTO

— — — — — — — — —

3. ROSEUS

— — — — — —

a. Composed of simple squamous epithelium resting on a thin layer of areolar connective tissue

b. Lines body surfaces that open directly to the body's exterior

c. Lines some of the closed body cavities and covers many of the organs in those cavities

d. The body's largest membrane

e. Secretes a fluid to help prevent friction as the organs move

f. Consists of different types of epithelium, depending on the location and function of the membrane

g. Consists of a layer of epithelium resting on a layer of connective tissue

h. Secretes mucus

i. Consists of three types: pleural, pericardial, and peritoneal

Epithelial Membranes

Firm up your knowledge of epithelial membranes by coloring the structures in the figure as suggested:

- Outline the mucous membranes in pink.
- Outline the cutaneous membrane in yellow.
- Outline the visceral pleura in blue.
- Outline the parietal pleura in purple.
- Outline the peritoneal membrane in green.
- Outline the pericardial membrane in red.

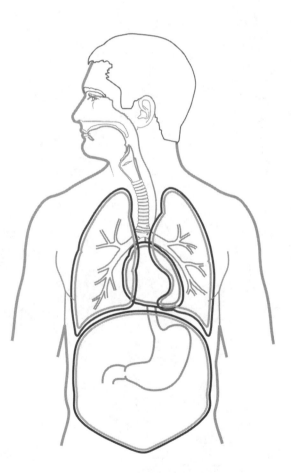

5

INTEGUMENTARY SYSTEM

The skin—which, together with the hair and nails, forms the integumentary system—is one of the largest organs in the body. Despite its thinness, it consists of multiple layers and many cell types. It also performs many functions crucial for homeostasis and even survival. Use the activities in this chapter to test yourself about this vital body system.

Conceptualize in Color: **Skin Structures**

Color these skin structures in the figure shown here. Use the colors suggested or choose your own.

- Epidermis: Brown
- Dermis: Pink
- Hypodermis: Yellow
- Eccrine sweat gland: Orange
- Apocrine sweat gland: Purple
- Sebaceous gland: Green

- Hair follicle: Light beige
- Hair bulb: Blue
- Hair shaft: Black
- Dermal papilla: Dark pink
- Arrector pili muscle: Red

Skin Structures

Complete the following crossword puzzle to strengthen your knowledge of skin structures and terms.

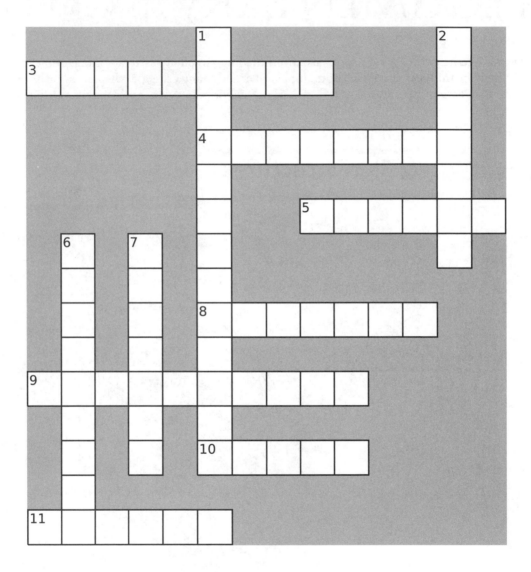

ACROSS

3. The skin is also called the _____ membrane.

4. Excessive hair loss

5. The inner, deeper layer of the skin

8. Outermost layer of the epidermis is called the stratum _____.

9. Inflammation of the skin characterized by itching and redness

10. Oily substance produced by sebaceous glands

11. Dead tissue resulting from a burn

DOWN

1. Flattened cells making up the skin's outermost layer

2. Substance that gives hair and skin its color

6. The outermost layer of the skin

7. Ear wax

Formation of New Skin Cells

Following are the various events in the formation of new skin cells. Using the spaces provided, order the events in the proper sequence by inserting numbers.

_____ **A.** Flattened, dead cells called keratinocytes arrive at the stratum corneum.

_____ **B.** Cells stop dividing and produce keratin, which replaces the cytoplasm and nucleus of the cell.

_____ **C.** Stem cells in the stratum basale undergo mitosis.

_____ **D.** The cells flatten and die.

_____ **E.** As new cells are produced, they push older cells upward.

Drawing Conclusions: # Skin Color

Fill in the blanks to test your knowledge about skin color. Then color the figure below using the instructions provided.

1. Melanocytes are scattered through the _____ layer of the epidermis.

2. These cells produce a substance called _____.

3. A person's skin color is determined by the amount, and type, of _____.

4. The _____ forms a cap over the top of the cell _____ to protect it from the _____ rays of the sun.

Color each of the structures in the figure shown here. Use the colors suggested or choose your own.

- Melanocyte: Green
- Keratinocytes: Tan
- Melanin granules: Red
- Cell nucleus: Orange

Skin Changes

Fill in the blanks to complete each of the following sentences. Choose from the words listed in the Word Bank.

ADRENAL	**BRONZING**	**MELANIN**	**RED**
ALBINISM	**CYANOSIS**	**PALLOR**	**ERYTHEMA**
BLUE	**JAUNDICE**	**YELLOW**	

1. A deficiency of oxygen in circulating blood gives skin a _____ tint, a condition called
    _____.

2. Impaired liver function may cause the skin to take on a _____ tone, a condition called
    _____.

3. A deficiency of hormones from the _____ gland causes the skin to become golden-brown in color, which is called _____.

4. A genetic lack of _____ results in extremely pale skin, white hair, and pink eyes, a condition called _____.

5. Decreased blood flow, such as from exposure to cold, emotional stress, or low blood pressure, produces
    _____.

6. Increased blood flow in dilated vessels close to the skin's surface makes the skin appear more
    _____ in color, which is called _____.

Functions of the Skin

Using the spaces provided, list five key functions of the skin.

1. _____
2. _____
3. _____
4. _____
5. _____

Thermoregulation

Complete the following sentences to test your understanding of how the skin helps the body maintain a stable temperature. Choose from the words listed in the Word Bank.

CONSTRICT	**EVAPORATION**	**NERVES**	**SWEATING**
DILATE	**INCREASES**	**REDUCES**	

1. The skin contains _____ to cause blood vessels in the skin to dilate or constrict to regulate heat loss.

2. When chilled, the blood vessels _____; this _____ blood flow through the skin and conserves heat.

3. When overheated, the blood vessels in the skin _____; this _____ the flow of blood and increases heat loss.

4. If the body is still overheated, the brain stimulates _____; this results in _____ and cooling occurs.

Nail Changes

Highlight the correct word in each of the following sentences.

1. A condition in which the distal ends of the fingers enlarge, making them look like a drumstick, is called (clubbing)(breaking); it typically results from long-term (iron)(oxygen) deficiency.

2. One of the first signs of oxygen deficiency is when the nail beds appear (dark red)(blue).

3. Flattened or concave nail beds may indicate a deficiency of (protein)(iron).

4. Anemia may cause the nail beds to look (pale)(cyanotic).

5. Dark lines beneath the nail may indicate (melanoma)(basal cell carcinoma).

Unscramble the following words to discover the names of four types of skin glands. Then draw a line to link each gland with its particular characteristics.

1. RICEECN

   _ _ _ _ _ _ _

2. CANOERIP

   _ _ _ _ _ _ _ _

3. BECAUSESO

   _ _ _ _ _ _ _ _ _

4. CURIOUSMEN

   _ _ _ _ _ _ _ _ _ _

a. Contains a duct that empties onto the skin's surface

b. Produces ear wax

c. Contains a duct that empties sweat onto a hair follicle

d. Begin to function at puberty

e. Secretes an oily substance onto the hair follicle

f. Located mainly in the axillary and anogenital region

g. Secretion has a mild antifungal effect

h. Are widespread throughout the body but are especially abundant on the palms, soles, forehead, and upper torso

i. Excess secretions may accumulate in gland ducts, leading to pimples and blackheads

j. Produce sweat to help the body maintain a constant core temperature

k. Are scent glands that respond to stress and sexual stimulation

Just the Highlights: **Burns**

Highlight in yellow the sentences that pertain to first-degree burns, the sentences that pertain to second-degree burns in orange, and the sentences that pertain to third-degree burns in pink.

1. Known as a partial-thickness burn, this burn only involves the epidermis.

2. This burn results in blisters, severe pain, and swelling.

3. This burn often results from sunlight.

4. Because nerve endings have been destroyed, this burn may not be painful initially.

5. Known as a full-thickness burn, this burn extends through the epidermis and dermis and into the subcutaneous tissue.

6. This burn, known as a partial-thickness burn, involves the epidermis and part of the dermis.

7. This burn results in redness, slight swelling, and pain.

8. This burn often requires skin grafts.

6

BONES & BONE TISSUE

The bones forming the human skeleton are dynamic living tissue. Besides providing the framework of the body, bones generate blood cells, regulate blood calcium levels, and join with the muscular system to allow us to move. The activities in this chapter should help you refine your knowledge of both the form and function of this vital tissue.

Make a Connection: **Bone Classifications**

Unscramble the following words to discover the four categories of bones. Then draw a line to link each category to its specific characteristics.

1. GLON

— — — —

2. STROH

— — — — —

3. TLAF

— — — —

4. ARULERRIG

— — — — — — — — —

a. Serve to protect organs

b. Tend to be shaped like cubes

c. Are longer than they are wide

d. Come in various sizes and shapes

e. Work like levers to move limbs

f. Are thin and often curved

g. Are often clustered in groups

h. Examples include the femur of the thigh and the humerus of the arm

i. Are about as broad as they are long

j. Examples include the carpal bones of the wrist

k. Examples include the skull and the ribs

l. Examples include the vertebrae and facial bones

ACROSS

4. Disease meaning "porous bones"
6. Process by which bone cells destroy old bone and deposit new bone
7. Bone cells that dissolve unwanted or unhealthy bone
9. Bone found in the ends of long bones and the centers of most other bones
10. Mature bone cells that have become entrapped in the hardened bone matrix
11. Name for bone tissue
12. Break in a bone

DOWN

1. Type of marrow that produces blood cells
2. Process whereby fetal skeleton becomes bone
3. Substance from which most bones evolve
4. Bone cells that help form bone
5. Type of bone that forms the shafts of long bones and surrounds outer surfaces of other bones
8. Latticework of bone that makes up spongy bone

Color these parts of the long bone in the following figure. Use the colors suggested or choose your own.

1. Articular cartilage: Blue

2. Bone marrow: Yellow

3. Medullary cavity: Gold

4. Periosteum: Tan

5. Epiphyseal line: Brown

6. Draw a red line along the endosteum

7. Draw a bracket around each epiphysis

8. Draw a bracket around the diaphysis

Cancellous Bone

Color the following parts of cancellous (spongy) bone. Use the colors suggested or choose your own.

- Periosteum: Brown
- Compact bone: Gold
- Trabeculae: Yellow

Fill in the Gaps: **Compact Bone**

Fill in the blanks to complete the following sentences. Choose from the words listed in the Word Bank.

| BLOOD VESSELS | LACUNAE | NERVES | OSTEON |
| HAVERSIAN | LAMELLAE | OSTEOCYTES | VOLKMANN'S |

1. In compact bone, layers of matrix are arranged in concentric rings called _____ around a central _____ canal. This basic structural unit is called an _____.

2. _____ and _____ run through the center of the canal.

3. Tiny gaps between the rings, called _____, contain _____.

4. Transverse passageways called _____ canals transport blood and nutrients from the bone's exterior to the living cells inside.

Using the following figure, color red all the bones, or portions of bones, containing red bone marrow.

List for Learning: Bone Functions

Using the blank spaces, list seven functions of bone.

1. _____

2. _____

3. _____

4. _____

5. _____

6. _____

7. _____

Describe the Process: Ossification

Using the following figures as a guide, describe each step in the process of endochondral ossification.

Cartilage model
Step 1

Ossifying cartilage
Epiphysis
Diaphysis
Bone formation
Step 2

Marrow cavity
Primary ossification center
Blood vessel
Step 3

Marrow cavity
Blood vessel
Step 4

Step 1: _____

_____

Step 2: _____

_____

Step 3: _____

_____

Step 4: _____

_____

Highlight the correct word or phrase that makes each of the following statements true.

1. After birth, bone lengthening occurs at the (epiphyseal plate)(epiphyseal line).

2. (Articular)(Hyaline) cartilage forms the (epiphyseal plate)(epiphyseal line).

3. When bone lengthening stops, (articular cartilage)(the epiphyseal plate) is replaced with (compact bone)(spongy bone).

4. Bone thickening and widening occurs (for a fixed number of years)(throughout the life span).

5. The process by which old bone is destroyed and then replaced with new bone is called (remodeling)(ossification).

6. Physical exercise causes bones to (increase)(decrease) in density.

List for Learning: **Factors Affecting Bone Growth**

Using the spaces provided, list four factors that affect bone growth and maintenance.

1. _____

2. _____

3. _____

4. _____

Using the spaces provided, draw a bone that illustrates the types of fractures listed below. Then fill in the blanks in each sentence to correctly describe each fracture. **Hint:** *Some blanks require more than one word.*

A. Simple fracture

In this type of fracture, the skin and tissue near the fracture is _____.

B. Compound fracture

In this type of fracture, the skin near the site has been _____.

C. Greenstick fracture
This type of fracture usually
occurs in _____ .

D. Comminuted fracture
This type of fracture is often the result
of a _____ .

E. Spiral fracture
This type of fracture results
from a _____ .

Fracture Repair

In the following figures, color the stages in fracture repair. Use the colors suggested or choose your own.

- Hematoma: Red
- Soft callus: Pink
- Hard callus: Yellow
- Remodeled bone: Tan

Then, using the figures as a guide, describe each step in the fracture repair process.

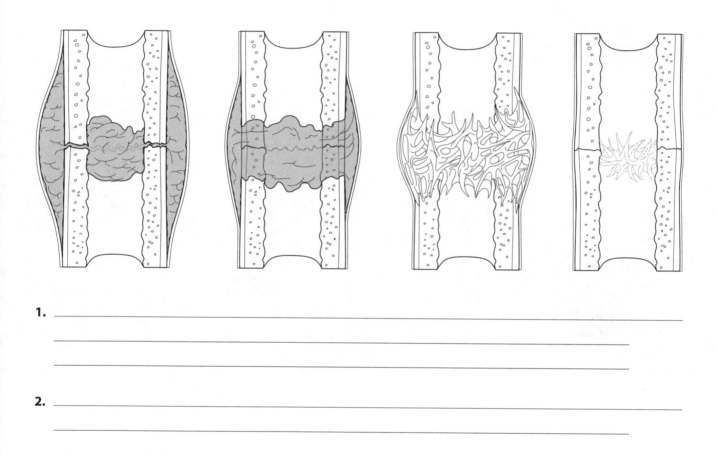

1. _____
   _____
   _____
   _____

2. _____
   _____
   _____

3. _____
   _____
   _____
   _____

4. _____
   _____

7

SKELETAL SYSTEM

Learning the names of the body's 206 bones, not to mention their locations and landmarks, can prove challenging. Completing the activities in this chapter, however, should help you do just that.

Just the Highlights: The Skeleton

In the following list, highlight the bones of the axial skeleton in one color (such as yellow) and the bones of the appendicular system in another color (such as blue).

1. Skull

2. Femur

3. Ribs

4. Clavicles

5. Vertebrae

6. Radius

7. Os coxae

8. Sacrum

9. Shoulder girdle

10. Mandible

Bone Surface Markings

Test your knowledge of the common terms used to describe bone surface markings by completing the following crossword puzzle.

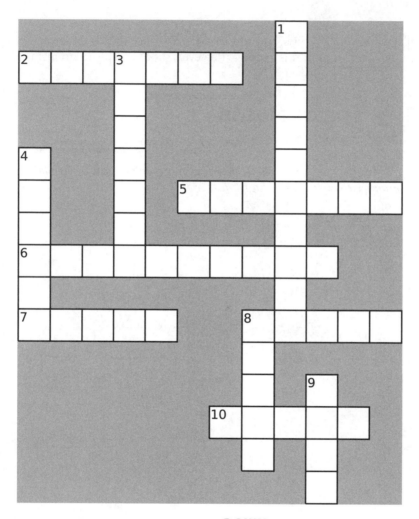

ACROSS

2. A projection or raised area

5. A round opening; usually a passageway for vessels and nerves

6. A rough, raised bump, usually for muscle attachment

7. A cavity within a bone

8. A moderately raised ridge

10. A flat surface

DOWN

1. A large process found only on the femur

3. A rounded knob; usually fits into a fossa on another bone to form a joint

4. A tube-like opening

8. A tunnel through a bone

9. The prominent, expanded end of a bone

The Skull

Color these bones of the skull in the figure below. Use the colors suggested or choose your own.

- Frontal bone: Orange
- Parietal bone: Blue
- Temporal bone: Green

- Occipital bone: Yellow
- Sphenoid bone: Red
- Ethmoid bone: Purple

More Bones of the Skull

Fill in the blanks with the proper word or words to complete each sentence. Choose from the words listed in the Word Bank.

ETHMOID	**MASTOID**	**SPHENOID**
EXTERNAL AUDITORY MEATUS	**NASAL CAVITY**	**SPINAL CORD**
FORAMEN MAGNUM	**SELLA TURCICA**	**ZYGOMATIC ARCH**

1. The _____ bone forms a key part of the cranial floor as well as the floor and side walls of the orbits. On top of that bone is an indented area called the _____ _____ , which houses the pituitary gland.

2. The top of the _____ bone is called the cribriform plate; it forms part of the roof of the _____ _____ .

3. The temporal bone contains an opening into the ear, which is called the _____ _____ _____ .

4. A prominent lump behind the ear is the _____ process of the temporal bone.

5. The cheekbone is called the _____ _____ .

6. The base of the skull contains a large opening called the _____ _____ through which the _____ _____ passes.

Unscramble the words in the left column below to discover the names of the four cranial sutures. Then draw a line to link each suture to its location.

1. RANLOCO

— — — — — — —

2. ATLASGIT

— — — — — — — —

3. QUASUMSO

— — — — — — — —

4. ABALDLIMOD

— — — — — — — — — —

a. The line of articulation between the parietal bones and the occipital bone

b. The joint between the parietal bones and the frontal bone

c. The joint between the right and left parietal bones

d. The line of articulation that runs along the top edge of the temporal bone

Facial Bones

Test your knowledge of the facial bones by coloring the following bones in the figure below. Use the colors suggested or choose your own.

- Mandible: Blue
- Maxillae: Green
- Zygomatic bones: Purple
- Lacrimal bones: Red

- Nasal bones: Yellow
- Inferior nasal conchae: Orange
- Vomer: Brown

Identify the various paranasal sinuses by coloring them in the following figure. Use the colors suggested or choose your own.

- Frontal sinuses: Yellow
- Maxillary sinuses: Blue

- Ethmoid sinuses: Pink
- Sphenoid sinus: Orange

Infant Skull

Solidify your knowledge of the infant skull by coloring the features of the skull. Then fill in the blanks of the sentences to identify some conditions that can cause changes in the fontanels.
Color these features in the following figure. Use the colors suggested or choose your own.

- Anterior fontanel: Pink
- Posterior fontanel: Blue
- Sagittal suture: Yellow

- Lambdoid suture: Green
- Squamous suture: Purple
- Coronal suture: Red

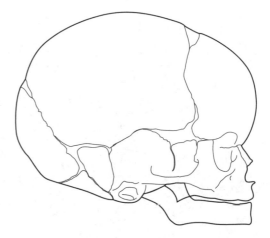

1. A bulging anterior fontanel signals increased _____ _____.

2. A sunken anterior fontanel suggests _____.

3. _____ causes the suture lines to widen abnormally.

In the figure below, color each of the following structures a different color: the cervical vertebrae, the thoracic vertebrae, the lumbar vertebrae, the sacrum, and the coccyx. Draw lines indicating the cervical curve, the thoracic curve, the lumbar curve, and the sacral curve.

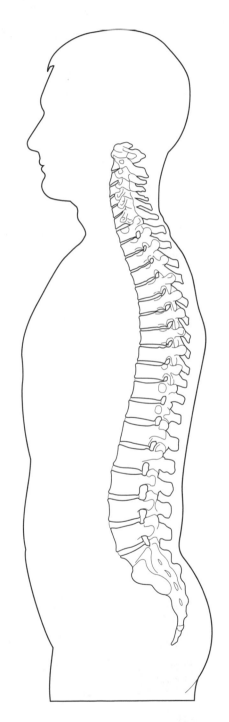

Hone your knowledge of vertebrae by coloring each of these structures in the following figure. Use the colors suggested or choose your own.

- Body: Purple
- Spinous process: Yellow
- Transverse process: Tan

- Lamina: Brown
- Vertebral foramen: Outline in blue

Thoracic Cage

Color each of these structures of the thoracic cage in the following figure. Use the colors suggested or choose your own.

- Manubrium: Brown
- Body of the sternum: Tan
- Xiphoid process: Pink
- True ribs: Blue

- False ribs: Yellow
- Floating ribs: Green
- Draw a red line at the suprasternal notch
- Draw a purple line at the costal margins

Test your knowledge of the bones of the pectoral girdle by first coloring the structures listed below. Use the colors suggested or choose your own. Then fill in the blanks in the sentences to describe their function.

- Scapula: Light tan
- Clavicle: Yellow
- Acromion process: Brown

- Coracoid process: Dark tan
- Glenoid cavity: Outline in pink

1. The acromion process articulates with the _____; it is the only point where the _____ and _____ attach to the rest of the skeleton.

2. The coracoid process provides a point of attachment for _____.

3. The glenoid cavity articulates with the head of the _____.

Color the bones of the arm as described below. Use the colors suggested or choose your own. Then identify key markings of those bones by writing the name of each marking in the appropriate space.

- Humerus: Brown
- Radius: Yellow
- Ulna: Pink

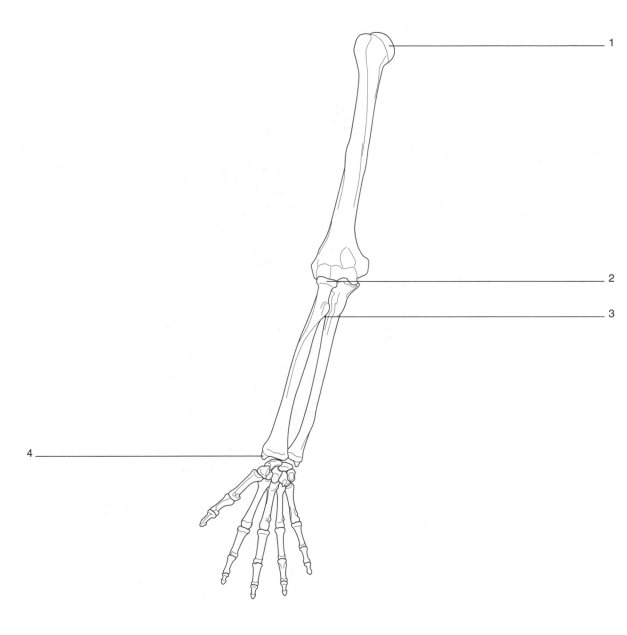

1

2

3

4

Improve your knowledge of the bones of the hand by coloring the following structures in the figure below. Use the colors suggested or choose your own. Then label each digit with the correct Roman numeral.

- Carpal bones: Blue
- Metacarpal bones: Pink
- Proximal Phalanges: Yellow

- Middle Phalanges: Orange
- Distal Phalanges: Green

Pelvic Girdle

Color the following structures in each os coxae, which together form the pelvic girdle. Use the suggested colors or choose your own.

- Ilium: Yellow
- Ischium: Orange
- Pubis: Pink
- Symphysis pubis: Blue

- Acetabulum: Green
- Iliac crest: Outline in Red
- Obturator foramen: Outline in Purple

Illuminate the Truth: **The Pelvis**

Highlight the word or phrase that makes each statement correct.

1. The (false pelvis)(true pelvis) extends between the outer, flaring edges of the iliac bones.
2. The (false pelvis)(true pelvis) extends between the pelvic brim.
3. The lower edge of the true pelvis is known as the (lesser pelvis)(pelvic outlet).
4. The distance between the two (ischial)(iliac) bones determines the pelvic outlet.
5. In males, the true pelvis is (deep and narrow)(wide and shallow).
6. Females have a pubic arch that is (narrower)(wider) than in males.
7. Females also have a (larger)(smaller) pelvic outlet.

Color the femur shown here using a color or colors of your choosing. Then identify key markings on the femur by writing the name of each marking in the appropriate space.

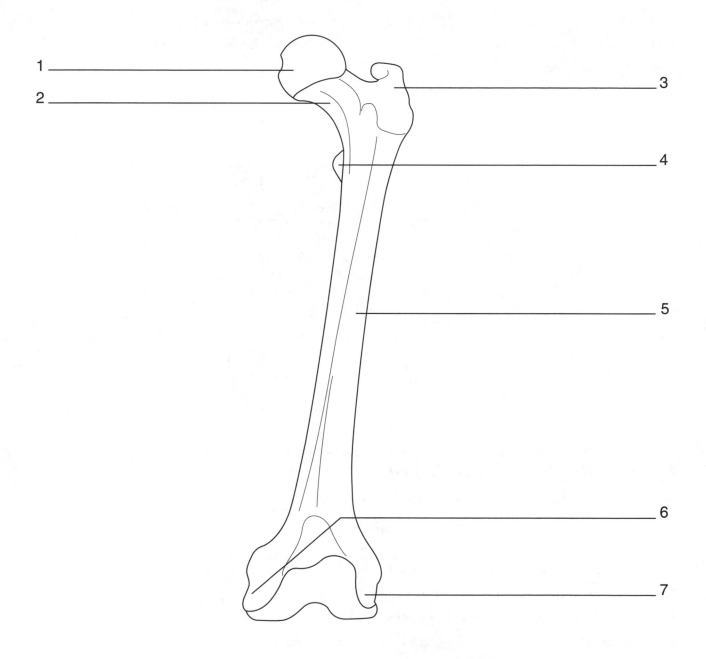

1 _____

2 _____

3 _____

4 _____

5 _____

6 _____

7 _____

Color the bones of the lower leg listed below. Use the colors suggested or choose your own. Then identify key landmarks by writing the name of each landmark in the appropriate space.

- Patella: Brown
- Tibia: Yellow
- Fibula: Pink

1 _____

2 _____

3 _____

Identify the bones of the foot by coloring each one listed below. Use the colors suggested or choose your own. Then number the metatarsals by labeling each with the proper Roman numeral.

- Calcaneus: Green
- Talus: Pink
- Navicular: Orange
- Cuneiforms: Yellow

- Metatarsals: Blue
- Proximal phalanges: Purple
- Middle phalanges: Red
- Distal phalanges: Tan
- Cuboid: Light blue

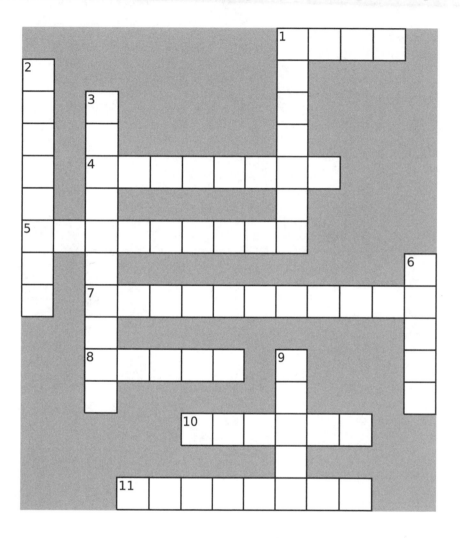

Puzzle It Out: Skeletal Facts

Continue to test your knowledge of the skeletal system by completing the following crossword puzzle.

ACROSS

1. Second cervical vertebra
4. Most frequently broken bone in the body
5. A lateral curvature of the spine
7. Procedure commonly performed following a herniated disc
8. Part of the body formed by the tarsal bones
10. The big toe
11. The gel-like core of the intervertebral disc is called the nucleus _____.

DOWN

1. A herniated disc results when the _____ fibrosus cracks.
2. An exaggerated thoracic curvature
3. The joint formed by the articulation of the os coxae with the sacrum
6. Bone in the neck that doesn't articulate with any other bone
9. The first cervical vertebra

8

JOINTS

Joints, or articulations, are the points where two bones meet. The body contains a number of different articulations, varying in both size and shape. It's these differences that allow us to perform a wide variety of movements, ranging from walking and running to writing or playing the piano.

Make a Connection: Classifications of Joints

Unscramble the following words to discover three classifications of joints. Then draw lines to the list on the right to link each joint classification to its characteristics.

1. VISAONLY

   — — — — — — — —

2. BIOSURF

   — — — — — — —

3. ANTISOCIALRUG

   — — — — — — — — — — — — —

a. Are freely movable

b. Result when bones are joined by cartilage

c. Result when collagen fibers from one bone penetrate the adjacent bone

d. The most numerous of the body's joints

e. Are slightly movable

f. Also called diarthroses

g. Are fixed joints

h. Also called amphiarthroses

i. An example is the symphysis pubis

j. Examples include the knee, hip, and elbow

k. An example is the suture joints in the adult skull

l. Also called synarthroses

Identify the key structures found in synovial joints by coloring the following figure. Use the colors suggested or choose your own colors.

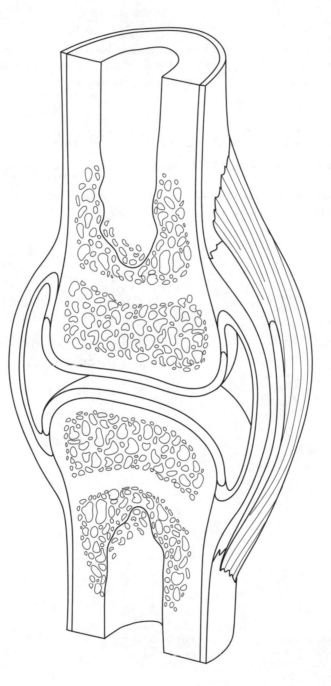

- Joint capsule: Green
- Synovial membrane: Purple
- Articular cartilage: Dark blue

- Ligaments: Gray
- Joint cavity: Light blue

Identify the type of synovial joint represented by each of the "hardware" joints. First, fill in the blanks to identify the type of joint, the movement the joint allows, and at least one location in the body where the joint can be found.

1.

- Type of joint: _____
- Movement: _____
- Location in the body:
  _____

2.

- Type of joint: _____
- Movement: _____
- Location in the body:
  _____

3.

- Type of joint: _____
- Movement: _____
- Location in the body:
  _____

4.

- Type of joint: _____
- Movement: _____
- Location in the body:
  _____

5.

- Type of joint: _____
- Movement: _____
- Location in the body:
  _____

6.

- Type of joint: _____
- Movement: _____
- Location in the body:
  _____

Movements of Synovial Joints

Describing the great variety of movements performed by synovial joints depends upon a specific vocabulary. Demonstrate your knowledge of these terms by writing the name of the movement being demonstrated by each of the following figures. Color the arrow signifying the direction of movement.

1. _____

2. _____

3. _____

4. _____

5. _____

6. _____

7. _____

8. _____

9. _____

10. _____

11. _____

12. _____

13. _____

14. _____

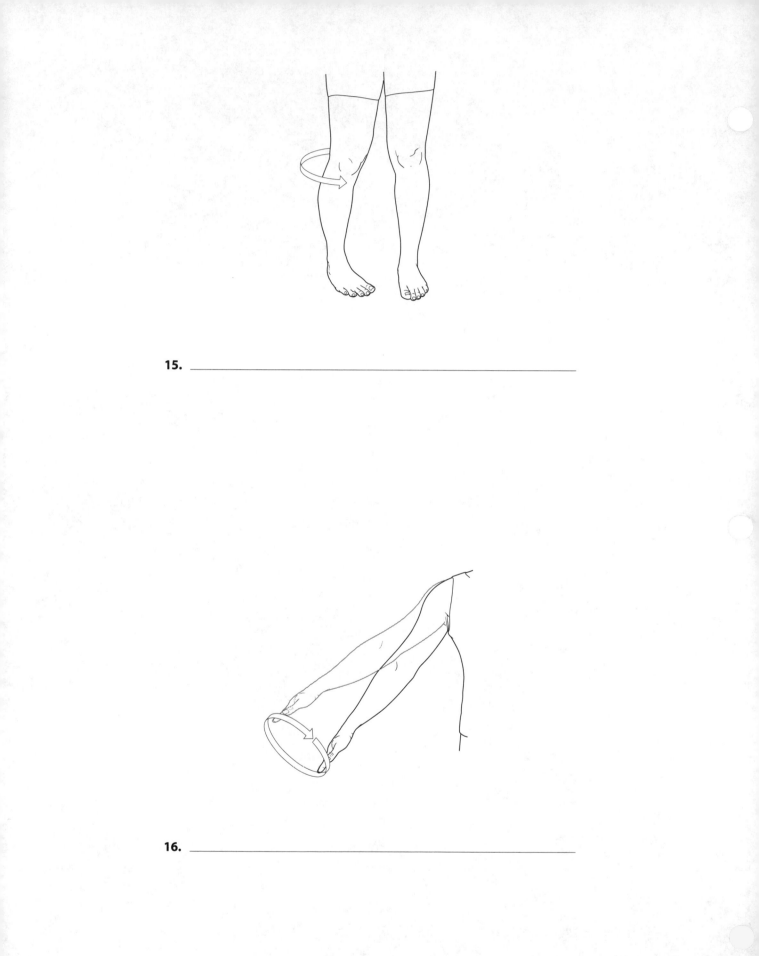

15. _____

16. _____

Identify the key structures of the knee by coloring the following figure. Use the colors suggested or choose your own colors.

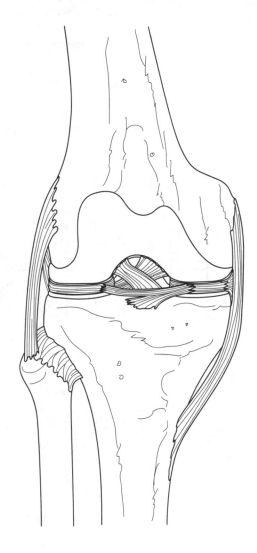

- Femoral condyles: Gray
- Medial meniscus: Light blue
- Lateral meniscus: Dark blue
- Posterior cruciate ligament: Orange

- Anterior cruciate ligament: Green
- Fibular collateral ligament: Tan
- Tibial collateral ligament: Brown

Test your general knowledge concerning joints by completing the following crossword puzzle.

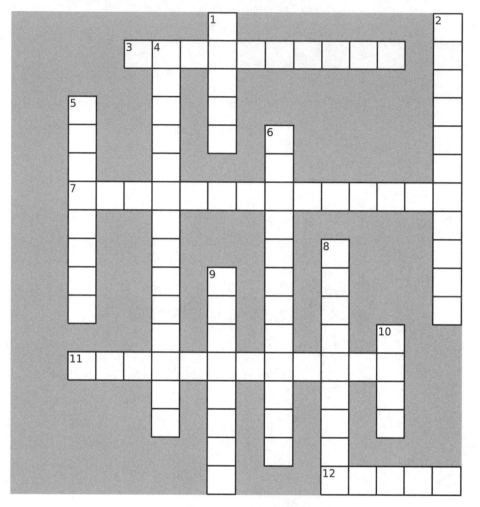

ACROSS

3. Type of arthritis that's an autoimmune disease
7. Type of arthritis attributed to the wear and tear of aging
11. Another name for a joint
12. Body joint consisting of two articulations

DOWN

1. Fluid-filled sac that resides in some joints
2. Type of surgical procedure often performed on the knee
4. The anterior cruciate ligament keeps the knee from doing this
5. Type of fluid that fills the joint capsule and lubricates the joint
6. Joint replacement
8. Meniscus is made of this material
9. Another name for the humeroscapular joint
10. Another name for the tibiofemoral joint

chapter

9
MUSCULAR SYSTEM

The body's more than 600 skeletal muscles give the body its shape and also allow it to move. Attached to bones, muscles produce movement through their ability to contract. Learning the names of key muscles and understanding the physiology behind movement can prove challenging. The activities in this chapter should help you master this important body system.

Make a Connection: Types of Muscles

*Unscramble the words on the left to discover the three types of muscle. Then draw a line linking each muscle type to its particular characteristics. (**Note:** Answers may be used more than once.)*

1. ACIDCAR

　— — — — — — —

2. MOSHTO

　— — — — — —

3. TALESELK

　— — — — — — — —

a. Found only in the heart

b. Does not appear striped, so it is called nonstriated

c. Consists of short, branching fibers that fit together at intercalated discs

d. Found in the digestive tract, blood vessels, and airways

e. Appears striped, or striated, when viewed under a microscope

f. Attached to bone and causes movement of the body

g. Known as involuntary muscle

h. Known as voluntary muscle

Test your knowledge of the various parts of a skeletal muscle by coloring the following structures in the figure below. Use the colors suggested or choose your own.

- Endomysium: Blue
- Perimysium: Yellow
- Epimysium: Red
- Fascia: Brown
- Draw a red circle around a single muscle fiber
- Draw a green circle around a fascicle

To reinforce your knowledge of the inner workings of a muscle, first fill in the blanks with the correct word or words. Then color each structure in the following figure; use the colors suggested or choose your own.

1. The membrane surrounding each fiber is called a _____.
    In the figure, color this structure pink.

2. Long protein bundles called _____ fill the sarcoplasm. These structures store

    _____ (which is used for energy) as well as oxygen.
    Color this structure yellow.

3. The smooth endoplasmic reticulum of a muscle fiber is called the _____;

    this is where _____ are stored.
    Color this structure blue.

4. A system of tubules called _____ allows _____
    to travel deep into the cell.
    Color these structures green.

5. Myofibrils consist of even finer fibers called _____.
    Color these structures brown.

Review the sliding-filament model of contraction by filling in the blanks in the following sentences. Then, in the space provided, draw two myofilaments: one displaying muscle relaxation and the second, muscle contraction.

1. Myofibrils consist of thin myofilaments (made of a protein called _____) and thick myofilaments (made of a protein called _____).

2. Myofibrils are arranged to form units called _____.

3. A plate or disc called a _____ is the anchor point for the thin myofilaments.

4. When a muscle begins to contract, the heads of the _____ myofilament latch onto the _____ myofilament, forming a _____.

5. The heads of the first myofilament then pull the second myofilament forward, shortening the _____ and pulling the _____ closer together.

Muscle Contraction

See if you can place the events that occur during muscle contraction and relaxation in their proper order. Insert numbers in the spaces provided to order the events in the proper sequence.

_____ **A.** An electrical impulse travels over the sarcolemma and inward along the T tubules, causing sacs in the sarcoplasmic reticulum to release calcium.

_____ **B.** The release of ACh stops and acetylcholinesterase breaks down any remaining ACh.

_____ **C.** Troponin and tropomyosin prevent the myosin heads from grasping the thin filament, and the muscle fiber relaxes.

_____ **D.** An electrical impulse causes small vesicles at the end of a motor neuron to bind with the cell wall and release the neurotransmitter acetylcholine (ACh).

_____ **E.** Calcium binds with the troponin on the actin filament, exposing attachment points.

_____ **F.** ACh diffuses across the synaptic cleft, where it stimulates receptors in the sarcolemma.

_____ **G.** Calcium ions are pumped back into the sarcoplasmic reticulum.

_____ **H.** The myosin heads of the thick filaments grab onto the thin filaments and muscle contraction occurs.

Test your knowledge of some of the terms associated with muscles by completing the following crossword puzzle.

ACROSS

1. Muscle that assists another muscle

3. A strong, fibrous cord that attaches muscle to bone

4. In _____ attachment, muscle fibers merge with the periosteum of the bone

6. The continuous state of partial muscle contraction is called muscle _____

8. A flat sheet of connective tissue that attaches a muscle to another muscle

10. A lack of ATP, such as occurs following death, causes muscles to become _____

11. Contraction in which the muscle changes length while the tension remains the same

12. The condition of rapid contraction with only partial relaxation is called incomplete _____

13. Contraction in which the tension within a muscle increases while its length remains the same

DOWN

1. The cytoplasm of a muscle cell

2. The connection between a motor neuron and a muscle fiber is called a _____ junction

5. Muscle that opposes the action of a prime mover

7. The process by which an increasing number of motor units are called into action, increasing the force of contraction

9. A single, brief contraction resulting when a muscle fiber receives a stimulus at or above threshold

How Muscles Are Named

Using the spaces provided, list the six characteristics of muscles that form the basis for muscle names.

1. _____

2. _____

3. _____

4. _____

5. _____

6. _____

Strengthen your knowledge of the muscular system by completing the following crossword puzzle.

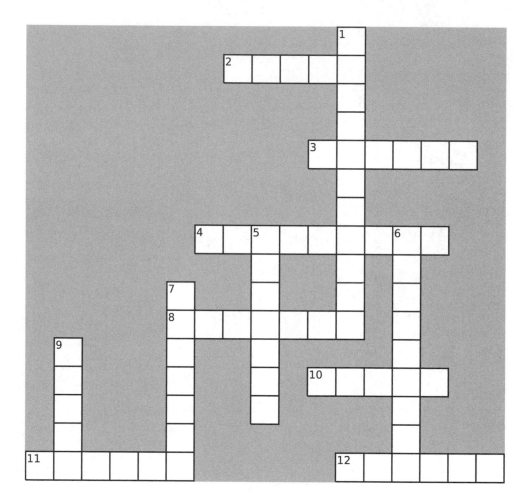

ACROSS

2. Thick midsection of a muscle
3. The end of a muscle that attaches to the more stationary bone
4. Type of muscle respiration that takes place without oxygen
8. Disuse causes a muscle to do this
10. At rest, muscles obtain most of their energy by metabolizing _____ acids.
11. Muscle term meaning shortest
12. Muscle term meaning longest

DOWN

1. Strength training causes a muscle to do this
5. Type of muscle respiration that uses oxygen
6. The muscle attachment that's more mobile
7. Muscle term meaning largest
9. Muscle term meaning small

Color the muscles in the figure shown here as described below; use the suggested colors or choose your own. Then link each muscle to its function by using the same color to highlight the sentence describing that muscle's action. For example, color the frontalis muscle brown; then, locate the sentence describing the action of the frontalis muscle and highlight it in brown.

Color the following muscles:

- Frontalis: Brown
- Orbicularis oculi: Pink
- Zygomaticus: Yellow
- Orbicularis oris: Orange
- Buccinator: Green
- Temporalis: Purple
- Masseter: Blue
- Sternocleidomastoid: Tan
- Trapezius: Red

Muscle function:

- Extends head when looking upward; elevates shoulder
- Closes eye when blinking or squinting
- Assists in smiling or blowing, such as when playing trumpet
- Aids in closing jaw
- Raises eyebrows when glancing upward or when showing surprise
- Closes mouth and purses lips, such as when kissing
- Closes jaw
- Flexes head downward; called "praying muscle"
- Draws mouth upward when laughing

Chapter 9 Muscular System **101**

Muscles of the Trunk

Color the muscles in the figure shown here as described below; use the colors suggested or choose your own. Next, link each muscle to its function by using the same color to highlight the sentence describing the muscle's action. For example, color the internal intercostals pink; then, locate the action of the internal intercostals in the list below and highlight it in pink.

Color the following muscles:

- External intercostals: Pink
- Internal intercostals: Red
- Diaphragm: Brown

Muscle function:

- Enlarges the thorax to trigger inspiration
- Elevate the ribs during inspiration
- Depress the ribs during forced exhalation

Color the muscles in the following figure as described below; use the colors suggested or choose your own. Next, link each muscle to its function by using the same color to highlight the sentence describing the muscle's action. For example, color the rectus abdominis pink; then, locate the sentence describing the action of the rectus abdominis and highlight it in pink.

Color the following muscles:

- Rectus abdominis: Pink
- Transverse abdominal: Yellow
- Internal oblique: Green
- External oblique: Purple
- Linea alba: Red

Muscle function:

- Compresses the contents of the abdomen
- Tough band of connective tissue; where the aponeuroses of muscles that form the abdominal wall meet
- Flexes the lumbar region of the spinal column to allow bending forward at the waist
- Stabilizes the spine and permits rotation at the waist
- Stabilizes the spine and aids in forceful expiration

Color the muscles in the following figures as described below; use the colors suggested or choose your own. Next, link each muscle to its function by using the same color to highlight the sentence describing the muscle's action. For example, color the deltoid muscle yellow; then, locate the sentence describing the action of the deltoid muscle and highlight it in yellow.

Anterior

Posterior

Color the following muscles:

- Deltoid: Yellow
- Pectoralis major: Green
- Serratus anterior: Pink
- Trapezius: Purple
- Latissimus dorsi: Blue

Muscle function:

- Raises and lowers shoulder
- Flexes and adducts upper arm, such as when hugging
- Abducts, flexes, and rotates arm, such as when swinging the arm (walking); also raises arm to perform tasks, such as writing on an elevated surface
- Pulls shoulder down and forward to drive forward-reaching and pushing movements
- Involved in activities such as swimming to adduct the humerus and extend upper arm backward

Color the muscles as instructed. Next, link each muscle to its function by using the same color to highlight the sentence describing the muscle's action . For example, color the brachialis pink; then, locate sentence describing the action of the brachialis muscle and highlight it in pink.

Color the following muscles:

- Brachialis: Pink
- Biceps brachii: Yellow
- Triceps brachii: Blue
- Brachioradialis: Green
- Pronator muscle: Purple
- Flexors: Orange

Muscle function:

- Prime mover when extending forearm
- Allows arm to pronate (palms down)
- Flexes wrist
- Prime mover when flexing forearm
- Assists with flexion of forearm
- Also assists with flexing forearm

Muscles Acting on the Hip and Thigh

Color the muscles in the following figures as described at the top of the facing page; use the colors suggested or choose your own. Next, link each muscle to its function by using the same color to highlight the sentence describing the muscle's action.

Color the following muscles:

- Iliacus: Red
- Psoas major: Green
- Sartorius: Dark blue
- Gracilis: Pink
- Adductor muscle group: Orange
- Gluteus maximus: Brown
- Gluteus medius: Yellow
- Hamstring group: Purple
- Quadriceps femoris: Light blue

Muscle function:

- Adducts thigh (two answers)
- Extends hip at thigh and flexes knee
- Prime mover for knee extension
- Flexes thigh (two muscles)
- Produces backswing of leg when walking; powers climbing up stairs
- Abducts and rotates thigh outward
- Aids in sitting cross-legged

List for Learning: Quadriceps Femoris

List the four muscles comprising the quadriceps femoris.

1. _____
2. _____
3. _____
4. _____

List for Learning: Hamstring Group

List the three muscles comprising the hamstrings.

1. _____
2. _____
3. _____

Muscles of the Lower Leg

*Color the muscles in the following figure as described below; use the colors suggested or choose your own. Next, link each muscle to its function by using the same color to highlight the sentence describing the muscle's action. (**Hint:** One muscle is used more than once.)*

Color the following muscles:

- Gastrocnemius: Green
- Soleus: Pink
- Calcaneal (Achilles) tendon: Yellow
- Tibialis anterior: Purple
- Extensor digitorum longus: Blue

Muscle function:

- Causes dorsiflexion of foot
- Extends toes and turns foot outward; also causes dorsiflexion of foot
- Cause plantar flexion (two muscles)

10
NERVOUS SYSTEM

The nervous system oversees and coordinates the activities of all of the body's systems. It receives millions of signals each day about changes within the body as well as the external environment. It processes that information, decides what actions need to occur, and then sends messages telling the various cells and organs how to respond. The nervous system is as complex as it is fascinating, and mastering its intricacies will require extra study. Doing the activities in this chapter will help.

Make a Connection: Cells of the Nervous System

Unscramble the words on the left to discover the names of nervous system cells. Then draw a line to link each cell to its characteristics. (Note: Some cells have more than one characteristic listed.)

1. DECODELYINGROOT

   _ _ _ _ _ _ _ _ _ _ _ _ _ _ _

2. DEPLANEMY LECL

   _ _ _ _ _ _ _ _ _ _ _ _ _

3. CIGARLIMO

   _ _ _ _ _ _ _ _ _

4. WASHCNN CLEL

   _ _ _ _ _ _ _ _ _ _ _

5. CASTERTOY

   _ _ _ _ _ _ _ _ _

a. Provide structural support in the central nervous system

b. Some secrete cerebrospinal fluid

c. Form myelin sheath in the brain and spinal cord

d. Engulf microorganisms and cellular debris

e. Form myelin sheath around nerves in the peripheral nervous system

f. Line spinal cord and cavities of the brain

g. Help form blood–brain barrier

Complete the following crossword puzzle to review some of the basics about the nervous system.

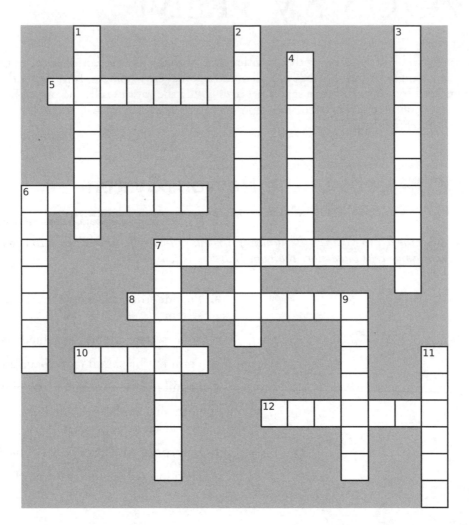

ACROSS

5. Another name for sensory neurons
6. Type of neuron that detects stimuli and transmits impulses to the brain and spinal cord
7. Essential for an injured nerve to regenerate
8. Division of the nervous system that provides for the body's "automatic" activities
10. Type of neuron that relays messages from the brain to muscles or gland cells
12. Impulse conducting cells of the nervous system

DOWN

1. Another name for motor neurons

2. Connect incoming sensory pathways with outgoing motor pathways in the CNS
3. The _____ nervous system consists of the network of nerves throughout the body
4. Division of the nervous system that carries signals from the organs
6. Division of the nervous system that carries impulses to and from skeletal muscles
7. Supportive cells of the nervous system
9. The _____ nervous system consists of the brain and spinal cord
11. Myelinated nerve fibers transmit impulses _____ than unmyelinated fibers

Improve your knowledge of neuron structure and function by filling in the blanks in the following sentences. Next, color the neuron using the colors suggested, or use your own colors.

1. The cell body, also called the _____,

   is the control center of the neuron and contains

   the _____.
   (Color the cell body blue.)

2. Dendrites receive signals from other _____

   and transmit the information _____ the
   cell body.
   (Color the dendrites green.)

3. The axon carries signals _____

   the cell body.
   (Color the axon yellow.)

4. Gaps in the myelin sheath are called _____

   _____.

   (Color these areas red.)

5. The synaptic knobs, which lie at the terminal

   point on each branch of the axon, secrete a

   _____.

   (Color the synaptic knobs brown.)

Describe the process of neural transmission by filling in the blanks in the following sentences. As you do, use the figures provided beneath each sentence to illustrate the process.

1. The phase in which the nerve is resting but has the potential to react if a stimulus comes along is called _____. In this phase, the inside of the cell has a _____ charge while the outside has a _____ charge. The interior is rich in _____ ions while the exterior is rich in _____ ions.

2. In depolarization, a stimulus causes _____ ions to enter the cell, and the interior changes from _____ to _____.

3. In _____ potential, the nerve becomes active and conducts an impulse along the axon. When this happens, more _____ ions enter the cell, and the nerve impulse continues down the axon.

4. In repolarization, _____ ions flow out of the cell. When this happens, the interior assumes a _____ charge while the exterior has a _____ charge.

_____

_____

4

5. During the _____ period, the neuron is polarized but won't respond to a stimulus until the sodium–potassium pump restores _____ ions to the outside of the membrane and _____ ions to the inside.

_____

_____

5

The transmission of an impulse from one neuron to the next follows a precise sequence of events. Use the spaces below to describe the numbered events in the illustration. Color the portion of the figure illustrating each step as you go along.

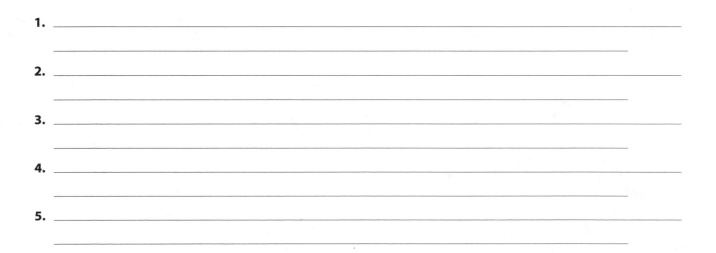

1. _____

_____

2. _____

_____

3. _____

_____

4. _____

_____

5. _____

_____

The Spinal Cord

Highlight the word or phrase that correctly completes each sentence.

1. The spinal cord extends from the base of the brain until about the (first lumbar vertebra)(last lumbar vertebra).

2. Extending from the end of the spinal cord is a bundle of nerve roots called the (cauda equina)(ganglion).

3. Gray matter appears gray because of its (abundance of myelin)(lack of myelin).

4. The (white matter)(gray matter) contains bundles of axons called tracts that carry impulses from one part of the nervous system to another.

5. The small space between the outer covering of the spinal cord and the vertebrae is called the (subdural space)(epidural space).

List for Learning: # Meninges

List the three layers of the meninges, starting with the innermost layer.

1. _____

2. _____

3. _____

Spinal Nerves and Meninges

Color the structures in the following figure. Use the colors suggested or choose your own.

- Dorsal nerve root: Green; insert a red arrow to depict the direction the impulse is traveling
- Ventral nerve root: Blue; insert a red arrow to depict the direction the impulse is traveling
- Ganglia: Yellow
- Spinal nerve: Orange
- Pia mater: Beige
- Dura mater: Purple
- Arachnoid mater: Pink
- Subarachnoid space: Dark blue
- Gray matter: Gray
- White matter: White

Differentiate between sensory and motor tracts by highlighting all the names and characteristics of sensory tracts in yellow and the names and characteristics of motor tracts in blue.

1. Ascending tracts

2. Descending tracts

3. Impulses travel down the spinal cord to skeletal muscles

4. Impulses travel up the spinal cord to the brain

5. Dorsal column (which relays sensations of deep pressure, proprioception, and vibration)

6. Extrapyramidal tracts (associated with balance and muscle tone)

7. Spinocerebellar tract (responsible for proprioception)

8. Corticospinal (responsible for fine movements of hands, feet, fingers, and toes)

9. Spinothalamic tract (relays sensations of temperature, pressure, pain, and touch)

10. Pyramidal tracts

Complete the following crossword puzzle to test your knowledge of some of the key terms related to spinal nerves.

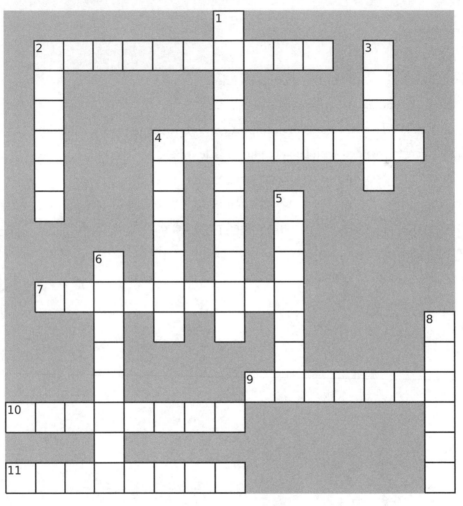

ACROSS

2. Paralysis of the legs resulting from a spinal cord injury between levels T1 and L1
4. Bundles of nerve fibers
7. Area innervated by a spinal nerve
9. Largest nerve in the body
10. Fibrous connective tissue that covers the spinal cord
11. Nerve susceptible to damage from improper use of crutches

DOWN

1. The crossing of spinal cord tracts from one side of the body to the other in the brainstem
2. A network of spinal nerves
3. Term used for nerves that carry both sensory and motor fibers
4. Key nerve of the lumbar plexus
5. Nerve that stimulates the diaphragm
6. Plexus that innervates the lower part of the shoulder and arm
8. Plexus formed from fibers from nerves L4, L5, and S1 through S4

Color the area innervated by cervical nerves blue, by thoracic nerves pink, by lumbar nerves orange, and by sacral nerves green.

Sequence of Events: **Somatic Reflex**

Insert the numbers 1 through 5 in the spaces provided to identify the sequence of events that occur in a somatic reflex.

_____ **A.** The motor neuron sends an impulse to a muscle.

_____ **B.** Somatic receptors detect a sensation.

_____ **C.** The impulse immediately passes to a motor neuron.

_____ **D.** Afferent fibers send a signal to the spinal cord.

_____ **E.** The muscle contracts.

Overview of the Brain

Highlight the correct word or phrase in the following sentences.

1. The largest portion of the brain is the (cerebrum)(cerebellum).

2. The structure residing deep inside the brain that contains the thalamus and hypothalamus is the (corpus callosum)(diencephalon).

3. The area of the brain that contains more neurons that the rest of the brain combined is the (cerebrum)(cerebellum).

4. The deep groove that divides the cerebrum into right and left hemispheres is the (corpus callosum)(longitudinal fissure).

5. The thick ridges covering the surface of the brain are called (sulci)(gyri).

6. The shallow grooves along the surface of the brain are called (sulci)(gyri).

7. (Gray matter)(White matter) covers the surface of the brain while (gray matter)(white matter) fills the interior.

8. Chambers inside the brain that are filled with cerebrospinal fluid are called (sinuses)(ventricles).

9. The bundle of nerves that connects the brain's two hemispheres is the (longitudinal fissure)(corpus callosum).

10. Patches of gray matter inside the brain are called (ganglia)(nuclei).

List for Learning: # The Brainstem

List the three structures that make up the brainstem.

1. _____

2. _____

3. _____

Identify key structures associated with the meninges by coloring each structure in the following figure. Use the colors suggested or choose your own.

- Dura mater: Pink
- Arachnoid mater: Orange
- Pia mater: Tan
- Dural sinus: Blue
- Arachnoid villi: Yellow
- Falx cerebri: Purple
- Draw a red line to identify the subdural space
- Draw a green line to identify the subarachnoid space
- Color the gray matter gray and the white matter either white or light gray

Trace the formation of cerebrospinal fluid (CSF) by placing the following events in the proper sequence: Insert the number 1 in the space by the first event, 2 by the second event, and so on. Then insert those same numbers in the accompanying figure to trace the flow of CSF. Color the ventricles and insert arrows to show the direction of flow.

_____ **A.** Some of the CSF flows through two tiny openings (foramina).

_____ **B.** The CSF is reabsorbed into the venous bloodstream by arachnoid villi.

_____ **C.** The choroid plexus in each lateral ventricle secretes CSF.

_____ **D.** The CSF flows through the subarachnoid space, up the back of the brain, down around the spinal cord, and up the front of the brain.

_____ **E.** The CSF flows into the third ventricle, where the choroid plexus adds more fluid.

_____ **F.** The CSF flows into the fourth ventricle, where a choroid plexus adds more CSF.

Unscramble the words on the left to discover the three components of the brainstem. Then draw lines to link each structure to its characteristics.

1. BRADMINI

_ _ _ _ _ _ _ _

2. SNOP

_ _ _ _

3. LADLEMU BOLOGNATA

_ _ _ _ _ _ _ _

_ _ _ _ _ _ _ _ _

a. Attaches brain to spinal cord

b. Contains centers for auditory and visual reflexes

c. Cranial nerves V (trigeminal), VI (abducens), VII (facial), and VIII (vestibulocochlear) arise here

d. Contains cardiac center (which regulates heart rate) as well as vasomotor center (which controls blood vessel diameter)

e. Contains two respiratory centers, which regulate breathing

f. Contains clusters of neurons integral to muscle control

g. Contains tracts that convey signals to and from different parts of the brain

---

Illuminate the Truth: **Brain Structures**

Test your knowledge of the various brain structures and their functions by highlighting the correct word or phrase in each of the following sentences.

1. The (cerebrum)(cerebellum) contains more neurons than any other portion of the brain.

2. The (hippocampus)(diencephalon) lies in the central portion of the brain and consists of several structures, including the thalamus and hypothalamus.

3. The (reticular activating system)(limbic system) is charged with maintaining a state of wakefulness.

4. The ability to think and use judgment is attributed to the (cerebellum)(cerebrum).

5. The thalamus is a gateway for nearly every (motor)(sensory) impulse traveling to the cerebral cortex.

6. Sometimes called the "emotional brain," the (hypothalamus)(limbic system) is the seat of emotion and learning.

7. The (amygdala) (hippocampus) converts short-term to long-term memory, making it crucial for memory and learning.

8. Cerebellar dysfunction often causes (stiffness and muscle pain)(poor balance and a spastic gait).

9. The (cerebral cortex)(hypothalamus) contains control centers for hunger, thirst, and temperature regulation.

10. The cerebrum is divided into five lobes by obvious (sulci)(gyri).

11. Two almond-shaped masses of neurons on either side of the thalamus, the (amygdala)(hippocampus) stores and can recall emotions from past events.

12. The hippocampus and amygdala are components of the (thalamus)(limbic system).

13. The surface of the cerebrum is called the (corpus callosum)(cerebral cortex).

14. The (hypothalamus)(hippocampus) controls the autonomic nervous system.

Drawing Conclusions: Cerebrum

Color the lobes of the cerebrum using the colors suggested below, or choose your own colors. Then, in the spaces provided, list some of the key functions of each lobe.

- Frontal lobe: Green
  Frontal lobe functions: _____
  _____

- Occipital lobe: Pink
  Occipital lobe functions: _____
  _____

- Parietal lobe: Blue
  Parietal lobe functions: _____
  _____

- Temporal lobe: Yellow
  Temporal lobe functions: _____
  _____

- Draw a red line along the central sulcus
- Draw a purple line along the lateral sulcus

Inside the Cerebrum

Color the structures in the figure below. Use the colors suggested or choose your own.

- Cerebral cortex: Gray
- Basal nuclei: Gray
- Corpus callosum: Blue
- Tracts in the brainstem: Green

Functional Areas of the Cerebral Cortex

Color the following areas of the cerebral cortex. Use the colors suggested or choose your own.

- Primary motor cortex: Dark blue
- Motor association area: Light blue
- Primary somatic sensory area: Dark green
- Somatic sensory association area: Light green
- Olfactory association area: Orange
- Primary auditory area: Red
- Auditory association area: Pink
- Primary visual cortex: Dark purple
- Visual association area: Light purple
- Primary gustatory complex: Yellow
- Wernicke's area: Brown
- Broca's area: Fuchsia

Functions of the Cerebral Cortex

Fill in the blanks with the correct word or phrase to identify the functions of specific areas in the cerebral cortex. Choose from the words listed in the Word Bank. (Hint: Not all the words will be used.)

ANGULAR GYRUS	**PRIMARY AUDITORY COMPLEX**
AUDITORY ASSOCIATION AREA	**PRIMARY GUSTATORY COMPLEX**
BROCA'S AREA	**PRIMARY VISUAL CORTEX**
LEFT	**RIGHT**
MOTOR ASSOCIATION AREA	**SOMATIC SENSORY ASSOCIATION AREA**
POSTCENTRAL GYRUS	**VISUAL ASSOCIATION AREA**
PRECENTRAL GYRUS	**WERNICKE'S AREA**

1. The _____ is the primary somatic sensory area, receiving impulses of heat, cold, and touch from all over the body.

2. The _____ is the area that allows us to pinpoint the location of pain, identify a texture, and be aware of how our limbs are positioned.

3. Neurons in the _____ determine which movements are required to perform a specific task.

4. Neurons in the _____ send impulses through the motor tracts in the brainstem and spinal cord to skeletal muscles to trigger movement.

5. The _____ is responsible for hearing, while the
_____ gives us the ability to recognize familiar sounds.

6. The _____ is responsible for sight while the
_____ interprets the visual information and allows us to recognize familiar objects.

7. _____ is responsible for language comprehension; an injury here affects one's ability to understand what others are saying.

8. _____ controls the muscle movements required for speech; an injury here will impair a person's ability to form words.

9. Because of decussation, the right side of the cerebral cortex receives signals from the _____ side of the body.

Write the name of each cranial nerve next to the Roman numeral representative of that nerve. Then draw a line to link each nerve to its characteristics. Some characteristics may link to more than one nerve, while other nerves may have more than one characteristic.

I _____

II _____

III _____

IV _____

V _____

VI _____

VII _____

VIII _____

IX _____

X _____

XI _____

XII _____

a. Mixed branch controls chewing and detects sensations in lower jaw

b. Links the retina to the brain's visual cortex; damage causes blindness in part or all of a visual field

c. Regulates voluntary movements of the eyelid and eyeball

d. Damage to sensory branch causes loss of sensation in upper face

e. Governs tongue movements, swallowing, and gagging

f. Damage causes tongue to deviate toward injured side

g. Damage here can cause a drooping eyelid and dilated pupil

h. Damage causes sagging facial muscles and distorted sense of taste

i. Longest and most widely distributed cranial nerve

j. Concerned with hearing and balance

k. Plays a key role in many heart, lung, digestive, and urinary functions

l. Controls movement in the head, neck, and shoulders

m. Ophthalmic branch triggers corneal reflex

n. Governs sense of smell

o. Damage causes deafness, dizziness, nausea, and loss of balance

Fill in the blanks in the following chart to compare these two divisions of the nervous system.

SOMATIC	AUTONOMIC
Innervates _____ muscle	Innervates _____, _____ muscle, and cardiac muscle
Consists of _____ nerve fiber leading from CNS to target (*Hint*: A number)	Consists of _____ nerve fibers that synapse at a _____ before reaching target
Secretes the neurotransmitter _____ _____	Secretes _____ and _____ as neurotransmitters
Has an _____ effect on target cells	Has an _____ or _____ effect on target cells
Operates under _____ control	Operates _____

Actions of Sympathetic and Parasympathetic Divisions

In the following list, highlight the effects of the sympathetic division in pink and those of the parasympathetic division in yellow.

1. Increases alertness

2. Increases heart rate

3. Constricts bronchial tubes to decrease air flow in lungs

4. Dilates bronchial tubes to increase air flow in lungs

5. Stimulates secretion of thick salivary mucus

6. Has a calming effect

7. Has no effect on blood vessels of skeletal muscles

8. Stimulates sweat glands

9. Stimulates intestinal motility and secretion to promote digestion

10. Causes "fight or flight" response

11. Has no effect on sweat glands

12. Has no effect on the urinary bladder or internal sphincter

13. Stimulates the bladder wall to contract and the internal sphincter to relax to cause urination

14. Stimulates adrenal medulla to secrete epinephrine

15. Causes the "resting and digesting" state

16. Dilates blood vessels of skeletal muscles to increase blood flow

17. Inhibits intestinal motility

Divisions of the Autonomic Nervous System

Unscramble the words on the left to discover the names of two divisions of the autonomic nervous system. Then draw lines to link each division with its characteristics.

1. ABATHROOMCURL

— — — — — — — — — — — — — —

2. RASCALAIRCON

— — — — — — — — — — — —

a. Another name for the sympathetic division

b. Employs mostly norepinephrine as a neurotransmitter

c. Originates in the brain and sacral region

d. Fibers leave brainstem by joining with cranial nerve III, VIII, IX, or X

e. Produces widespread, generalized effects

f. Ganglia lie in or near target organ

g. Has long preganglionic and short postganglionic fibers

h. Employs acetylcholine as a neurotransmitter

i. Arises from the thoracic and lumbar regions of the spinal cord

j. Ganglia lie in a chain alongside spinal cord

k. Produces local effects

l. Has short preganglionic and long postganglionic fibers

m. Another name for the parasympathetic division

Autonomic Nervous System Terms

Complete the following crossword puzzle to test your knowledge of some key terms associated with the autonomic nervous system.

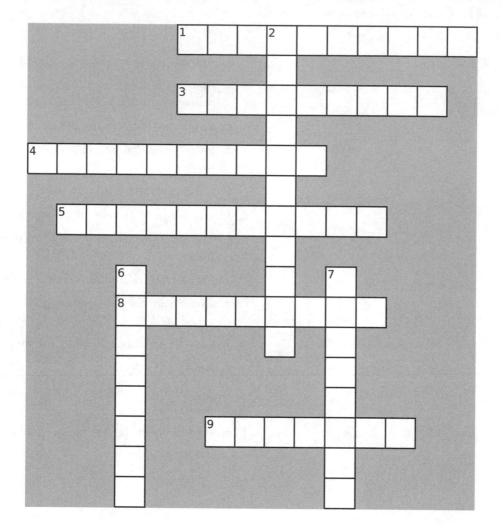

ACROSS

1. These receptors have a variable response to acetylcholine
3. These receptors are excited by acetylcholine
4. Fibers that secrete norepinephrine
5. The adrenal medulla secretes hormones that helps prolong the effects of this division of the autonomic nervous system
8. Beta-adrenergic receptors are _____ by norepinephrine
9. Alpha-adrenergic receptors are _____ by norepinephrine

DOWN

2. Fibers that secrete acetylcholine
6. The autonomic nervous system is sometimes called the _____ motor system
7. The effect of a neurotransmitter is determined mainly by the _____

Sympathetic and Parasympathetic Pathways

The two divisions of the autonomic nervous system employ two different neurotransmitters. After being released, neurotransmitters bind to different types of receptors. Test your knowledge of the neurotransmitters and receptors of the sympathetic and parasympathetic pathways by filling in the blanks in the following sentences. Choose from the words listed in the Word Bank. (Hint: Words may be used multiple times; also, some words may not be used at all.)

ACETYLCHOLINE (ACH)	**BETA-ADRENERGIC**	**NICOTINIC**	**TARGET ORGAN**
ADRENERGIC	**CHOLINERGIC**	**NOREPINEPHRINE (NE)**	
ALPHA-ADRENERGIC	**MUSCARINIC**	**RECEPTOR**	

1. The autonomic nervous system employs the neurotransmitters _____ and _____.

2. Fibers that secrete ACh are called _____ fibers; fibers that secrete NE are called _____ fibers.

3. The preganglionic fibers of both the sympathetic and parasympathetic divisions as well as the postganglionic fibers of the parasympathetic division are _____ fibers. They secrete the neurotransmitter _____.

4. Most of the postganglionic fibers of the sympathetic division are _____ fibers. They secrete the neurotransmitter _____.

5. ACh binds to _____ receptors and NE binds to _____ receptors.

6. The effect produced by a neurotransmitter is determined by the type of _____.

7. ACh may bind to either _____ receptors or _____ receptors.

8. All cells with _____ receptors are excited by ACh.

9. All cells with _____ receptors exhibit a variable response to ACh.

10. Cells with _____ receptors are excited by NE.

11. Cells with _____ receptors are inhibited by NE.

11

SENSE ORGANS

The sense organs allow us to see, hear, taste, and feel. These sensations not only allow us to derive pleasure from the environment, they also protect us from danger and contribute to our mental well-being. Complete the activities in this chapter to review this system.

List for Learning: Sensations

List the three kinds of information sensory receptors transmit about each sensation.

1. _____

2. _____

3. _____

List for Learning: Taste

See if you can list all five primary taste sensations.

1. _____

2. _____

3. _____

4. _____

5. _____

Terms of the Sensory System

Test your knowledge of some of the terms of the sensory system by completing the following crossword puzzle.

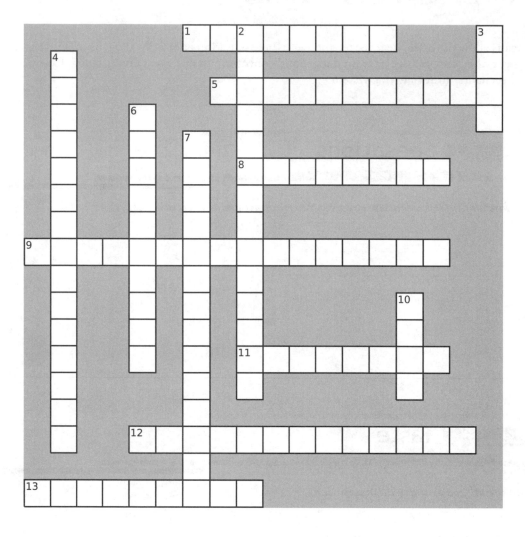

ACROSS

1. Protrusions of the tongue on which taste buds are located
5. Pain receptors
8. Pain originating in a deep organ that's sensed on the body's surface
9. Receptors that respond to stretch
11. Specialized nerve cells that detect physical or chemical events outside the cell membrane
12. Receptor that allows you to orient your body in space
13. Drug used to relieve pain

DOWN

2. Receptors found only in the eyes
3. Type of pain fiber that produces sharp, localized pain
4. Receptors activated by a change in temperature
6. When a stimulus is continuous, the firing frequency of the nerve begins to slow, causing the sensation to diminish; this is known as _____.
7. Receptors that react to odors
10. Type of pain fiber found on deep body organs

Review each step in the body's main pain pathway by filling in the blanks in the following sentences. As you go along, insert arrows in the figure to identify the pathway. Then color the key structures in the figure as desired.

1. Injured tissues release several chemicals that stimulate the _____ and trigger pain.

2. A neuron conducts a pain signal to the _____ horn of the spinal cord and then up the _____ tract to the _____ .

3. At the same time, the _____ tract carries pain signals to the reticular formation of the _____ .

4. The thalamus relays the signal from the _____ tract to the _____ _____ of the _____ . At that point, the person becomes aware of the pain.

5. The impulse from the spinoreticular tract bypasses the _____ and travels to the _____ and _____ system. These areas trigger _____ and _____ responses to pain, such as fear and nausea.

Sense of Smell

*Fill in the blanks to describe how the sense of smell occurs. Choose from the words listed in the Word Bank. (**Hint:** Not all the words will be used.)*

CILIA	**NASAL**	**PAPILLAE**
CRANIAL	**OLFACTORY**	**PRIMARY OLFACTORY**
ETHMOID	**OLFACTORY BULBS**	**SPHENOID**

1. Receptors for the sense of smell, called _____ receptors, are buried in the roof of the _____ cavity.

2. Incoming odor molecules bind to _____ projecting from the ends of the receptor cells.

3. This triggers a nerve impulse along nerve fibers leaving the nasal cavity through pores in the _____ bone.

4. The fibers synapse with other neurons in _____, a pair of structures underneath the brain's frontal lobe.

5. After being partially processed here, the signals continue to the _____ cortex in the brain.

Sections of the Ear

The ear has three sections: the outer ear, the middle ear, and the inner ear. In the following list, highlight the structures of the outer ear pink, the middle ear blue, and the inner ear yellow.

1. Eustachian tube
2. Bony labyrinth
3. Auricle
4. Vestibule
5. Auditory canal

6. Cochlea
7. Auditory ossicles
8. Tympanic membrane
9. Semicircular canals

Drawing Conclusions: **The Ear**

Improve your understanding of ear structures and functions by filling in the blanks in the following sentences. Color the structures as described in the figure below.

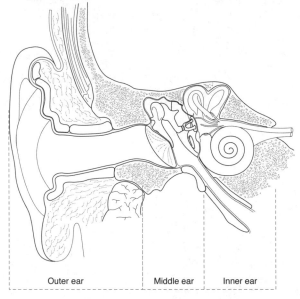

Outer ear   Middle ear   Inner ear

1. The _____ is the visible part of the ear. Its main function is to funnel _____ into the ear. (Color this part of the ear tan.)

2. The _____ leads through the temporal bone to the eardrum. Glands in this part of the ear secrete _____. (Outline this structure in red.)

3. The malleus, incus, and stapes are called the _____ _____; they connect the _____ to the _____ ear. (Color the malleus pink, the incus blue, and the stapes green.)

4. The stapes fits in the _____ window of the _____. (Outline this window in dark blue.)

5. The _____ _____ separates the outer ear from the middle ear. It vibrates in response to _____ _____. (Color this structure orange.)

6. The _____ tube is a passageway from the middle ear to the nasopharynx. Its purpose is to equalize _____ on both sides of the tympanic membrane. (Color this structure purple.)

7. The _____ _____ lie at right angles to each other and are crucial for the maintenance of balance. (Color this structure green.)

8. The _____ marks the entrance to the labyrinths and contains organs necessary for the sense of balance. (Color this structure light blue.)

9. The _____ is a snail-like structure that contains the organ of Corti. (Color this structure brown.)

10. The two nerves leading from the ear are the _____ nerve, which is linked to the vestibule, and the _____ nerve, which leaves from the cochlea. (Color these two nerves pink and yellow, respectively.)

Drawing Conclusions: How Hearing Occurs

The structures of the inner ear are essential for hearing. Test your knowledge of these structures by coloring them as described in the figure.

- Cochlear duct: Green
- Tectorial membrane: Orange
- Basilar membrane: Purple

- Hair cells on the organ of Corti: Yellow
- Cochlear nerve: Tan

Next, describe the process of hearing by completing the following sentences. Insert arrows into the figure to show the progression of sound waves.

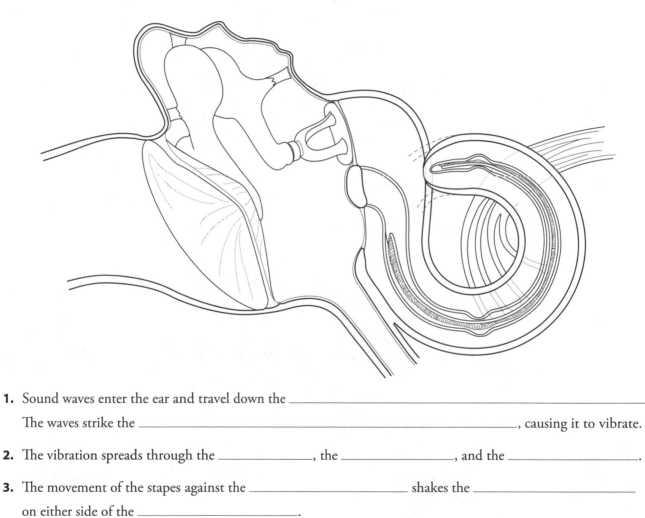

1. Sound waves enter the ear and travel down the _____.
   The waves strike the _____, causing it to vibrate.

2. The vibration spreads through the _____, the _____, and the _____.

3. The movement of the stapes against the _____ shakes the _____
   on either side of the _____.

4. The ripples in the _____ are transmitted through the roof of the _____
   to the _____. This causes nerve impulses to be transmitted along the
   _____ nerve. The impulses reach the _____ in the
   brain's _____ lobe, where it's interpreted as sound.

5. The ripples continue through the _____ and dissipate by striking the _____ window.

Accessory Eye Structures

Fill in the blanks in the following sentences to complete the information about key accessory structures of the eye. Then follow the instructions to color the structures in the figure.

1. The most significant role of the _____ is to enhance facial expression.
   (Color this structure black.)

2. The _____ protect the eye from foreign bodies and block light to allow for sleeping.
   (Color this structure pink.)

3. The thickened edge along the lower eyelid is called the _____ _____; it

   secretes _____ to slow the evaporation of tears.
   (Draw a black line along this structure.)

4. The _____ gland secretes _____ that flow onto the surface of the conjunctiva.
   (Color this structure blue.)

5. Tears drain through a tiny pore called the _____ _____.
   (Draw red dots at each of these locations.)

6. The passageway that carries tears into the nasal cavity is called the _____ duct.
   (Color this structure yellow.)

To enhance your knowledge of the anatomy of the eye, color the structures of the eye as instructed.

- Sclera: Tan
- Cornea: Light blue
- Iris: Green
- Ciliary body: Red
- Choroid: Brown
- Retina: Gold
- Optic nerve: Purple
- Part of the eye containing vitreous humor: Orange
- Part of the eye containing aqueous humor: Pink
- Lens: Gray

In each of the following sentences, highlight the word or phrase that correctly completes each sentence.

1. The opening between the eyelids is called the (palpebral fissure)(palpebrae).

2. The transparent mucous membrane lining the inner surface of the eyelid and most of the anterior surface of the eyeball is the (sclera)(conjunctiva).

3. Most of the muscles charged with moving the eyeball are innervated by the (facial nerve)(oculomotor nerve).

4. The (cornea)(sclera) is transparent tissue that sits at the anterior portion of the eye and admits light into the eye.

5. The (choroid)(ciliary body) secretes aqueous humor.

6. The (choroid)(sclera) supplies oxygen and nutrients to the retina and sclera.

7. The (oculomotor)(optic) nerve exits from the posterior portion of the eyeball.

8. Photoreceptors in the eye are located in the (cornea)(retina).

9. The center point of the retina when viewed through an ophthalmoscope is the (macula lutea)(fovea centralis).

10. The area that produces the sharpest vision is the (macula lutea)(fovea centralis).

11. Nerve fibers leave the retina at the (optic disc)(fovea centralis).

In the following figure, color the muscles as described.

- Superior oblique: Yellow
- Superior rectus: Blue
- Inferior oblique: Purple
- Inferior rectus: Green
- Medial rectus: Orange
- Lateral rectus: Pink

The Process of Vision

Describe how vision occurs by filling in the blanks in the sentences below and then carrying out the drawing activity described for each step.

1. Light rays entering the eye must be _____ so they focus on the retina. This process is

   called _____. The curved surface of the _____ allows much of this
   to happen.

(In the figure provided, insert lines and arrows to symbolize light rays entering the eye and focusing on the retina as described in the sentence above.)

2. The eyes also must be aligned so that the light rays from an object fall on the _____

   _____ of each retina. This is called _____.

(In the space provided below the figures, draw a set of eyeballs focusing on a distant object [the Statue of Liberty] and a second set of eyeballs focusing on a nearby object [the book]. Insert lines to signify light rays from the objects entering the eye and focusing on the retina.)

3. When focusing on a nearby object, the pupil _____. To accomplish this, the _____ _____ muscle constricts.

(Insert arrows into the figure below to illustrate this process.)

4. The opposite of this reaction is pupillary _____, which is accomplished when the _____ _____ muscle contracts.

(In the space beside the iris above, draw a second iris. Insert arrows to illustrate the process described here.)

5. To fine-tune for sharper focus, the lens also changes shape, a process called _____. When focusing on a distant object, the _____ muscle _____ and the lens _____.

(Illustrate this process using the figures provided. Insert light rays; also insert arrows to show the actions occurring within the eye.)

6. When focusing on a nearby object, the _____ muscle _____ and the lens _____.

(Illustrate this process using the figures provided. Insert light rays; also insert arrows to show the actions occurring within the eye.)

Unscramble the words on the left to discover the names of the photoreceptors of the eye. Then draw lines to connect each receptor to its characteristics.

1. DORS

   — — — —

2. NOSEC

   — — — — —

a. Concentrated in the center of the retina

b. Concentrated at the periphery of the retina

c. Active in dim light

d. Active in bright light

e. Responsible for color vision

f. Responsible for night vision

g. Cannot distinguish colors from each other

h. Primarily responsible for sharp vision

Just the Highlights: **Vision Neural Pathway**

The final step in the visual process involves relaying nervous impulses to the brain, where images are interpreted as sight. Highlight the correct word or phrase in each of the following sentences to identify the steps in the vision neural pathway.

1. Nerve impulses generated by the rods and cones leave the eye via the (optic)(oculomotor) nerve.

2. Nerve fibers from the nasal side (remain on the same side)(cross to the opposite side) of the brain at the (foramen magnum)(optic chiasm).

3. Nerve fibers on the temporal side (remain on the same side)(cross to the opposite side) of the brain at the (foramen magnum)(optic chiasm).

4. The impulses travel to the (primary visual cortex)(accessory visual cortex) in the (frontal)(occipital) lobe for interpretation.

Puzzle It Out: Eye Terms

Test your knowledge of terms relating to the eye by completing the following crossword puzzle.

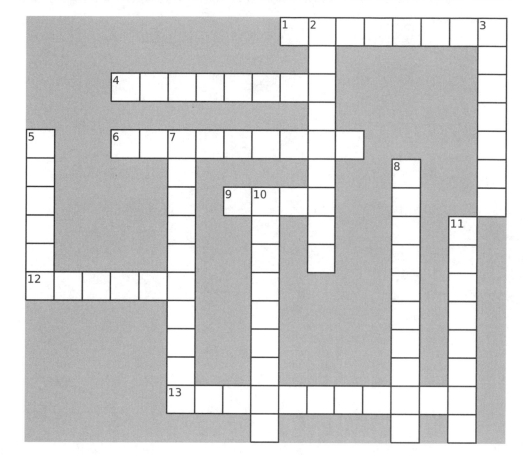

ACROSS

1. The jelly-like substance filling the posterior cavity is called _____ humor.
4. Clouding of the lens of the eye
6. Farsightedness
9. Eye structure that changes shape for near and far vision
12. Sharpness of vision is called visual _____.
13. Condition resulting from uneven curvature of the cornea

DOWN

2. Group of eye muscles arising from within the eye
3. Aqueous humor drains into the canal of _____.
5. Nearsightedness
7. Difficulty focusing on near objects due to a loss of lens flexibility as a result of aging
8. Normal vision
10. Group of eye muscles that move the eyeball
11. Condition caused by increased intraocular pressure

12
ENDOCRINE SYSTEM

Like the nervous system, the endocrine system promotes communication between cells, allowing them to coordinate and integrate their activities. Complete the exercises in this chapter to improve your knowledge of this important system.

Drawing Conclusions: Organs of the Endocrine System

Color each of the organs in the following figure. Write the name of the organ next to each number.

Review some general information about the endocrine system by completing the following crossword puzzle.

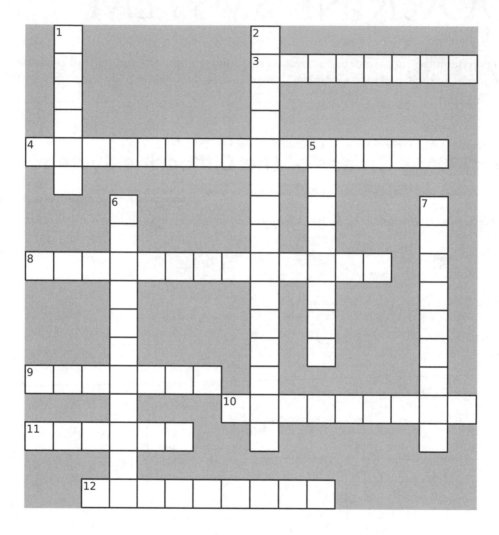

ACROSS

3. Endocrine glands are known as _____ glands.
4. Name for the posterior pituitary
8. Field of medicine that diagnoses and treats disorders of the endocrine system
9. Nonsteroid hormones are based on this substance.
10. Gland that exerts more influence over body processes than any other gland
11. Type of tissue making up the posterior pituitary
12. Type of tissue making up the anterior pituitary

DOWN

1. Cells having receptors for a particular hormone are called _____ cells.
2. Name for the anterior pituitary
5. Chemical messengers secreted by the endocrine system
6. Substance from which steroid hormones are made
7. Cells with more of these are more sensitive to a hormone's influence

Comparison of Endocrine and Nervous Systems

While both the endocrine and nervous systems work toward the same goal—homeostasis—their methods differ. In the following list, highlight the actions of the endocrine system in blue and the actions of the nervous system in yellow.

1. Employs hormones to relay messages

2. Secretes neurotransmitters into tiny space of a synapse

3. Adapts slowly to continual stimulation

4. Responds to stimuli quickly (milliseconds)

5. Exerts short-lived effects

6. Adapts quickly to continual stimulation

7. Responds slowly to stimuli (seconds to days)

8. Distributes hormones throughout the body via the bloodstream

9. Exerts long-lasting effects

10. Employs neurotransmitters to relay messages

Pituitary Gland Anatomy

Refine your knowledge of the anatomy of the pituitary gland by coloring the structures in the following figure. Use the colors suggested or choose colors of your own.

- Hypothalamus: Orange
- Anterior pituitary: Blue
- Posterior pituitary: Yellow
- Sphenoid bone: Brown
- Optic chiasm: Red
- Infundibulum: Pink

Anterior Pituitary

To understand the function of the anterior pituitary, fill in the blanks in the sentences, which are numbered to coordinate with the numbered structures in the illustration. Then follow the instructions to color the figure as described.

1. Neurons within the _____ synthesize various hormones that act on the anterior pituitary. Some of these hormones stimulate the anterior pituitary to secrete its hormones; these

   hormones are called _____ hormones. Others suppress hormone

   secretion by the anterior pituitary; these hormones are called _____ hormones.
   (In the figure, color the neurons yellow.)

2. These neurons release their hormones into a system of blood vessels called the _____

   _____ .
   (Color the structure described in this sentence light blue.)

3. From there, the blood travels straight to the _____ , where the
   hormones act on target cells. (Insert a series of small red dots to show the path traveled by the hormones.
   Insert small black arrows to show where the hormones are acting on target cells.)

4. This stimulates the _____ to release certain hormones into

   _____ .
   (Insert red arrows to show the release of the hormones.)

Hormones of the Anterior Pituitary

Test your knowledge about the hormones of the anterior pituitary by filling in the blanks in the following sentences. Choose from the list of words in the Word Bank.

ADRENOCORTICOTROPIC HORMONE (ACTH)	OVULATION
CARBOHYDRATES	PROGESTERONE
CORTICOSTEROIDS	PROLACTIN
ESTROGEN	SOMATOTROPIN
FOLLICLE-STIMULATING HORMONE (FSH)	SPERM
GROWTH HORMONE (GH)	TESTOSTERONE
LIPIDS	THYROID HORMONE
LUTEINIZING HORMONE (LH)	THYROID-STIMULATING HORMONE
MILK	THYROTROPIN

1. The thyroid gland is stimulated by _____ (also called _____) prompting it to secrete _____ .

2. The mammary glands are stimulated by _____ to secrete _____ .

3. The adrenal cortex is stimulated by _____ to secrete _____ .

4. _____ (also called _____) acts on the entire body to promote growth in bones and muscles and to metabolize _____ and _____ .

5. The secretion of the female hormones estrogen and progesterone is triggered by the release of _____ ; this same hormone stimulates _____ in females and the synthesis of the hormone _____ by the testes in males.

6. _____ stimulates the production of eggs in the ovaries of females and _____ in the testes of males.

Posterior Pituitary

Reinforce your knowledge of the function and hormones of the posterior pituitary by highlighting the word that correctly completes each sentence.

1. Unlike the anterior pituitary, which is composed of (glandular)(neural) tissue, the posterior pituitary is made of (glandular)(neural) tissue.

2. Nerve fibers forming the posterior pituitary originate in the (anterior pituitary)(hypothalamus).

3. Hypothalamic neurons (store)(synthesize) hormones, which they send down to the posterior pituitary to be (refined)(stored).

4. The posterior pituitary releases the hormones (continually)(when stimulated by the nervous system).

5. The hormones associated with the posterior pituitary are (somatotropin)(oxytocin) and (ACTH)(ADH).

Illuminate the Truth: **Thyroid, Parathyroid, and Pineal Glands**

Use a highlighter to illuminate the correct word or phrase in each of the following sentences.

1. The pineal gland produces (melatonin)(calcitonin), a hormone that rises (at night)(during the day) to trigger (alertness)(sleepiness).

2. The thyroid gland secretes (thyroid-stimulating hormone)(thyroid hormone), which (suppresses)(boosts) the body's metabolic rate.

3. The two lobes of the thyroid are connected by the (isthmus)(infundibulum).

4. The parathyroid glands are located on the (anterior)(posterior) side of the thyroid.

5. The parathyroid glands secrete parathyroid hormone in response to low levels of (thyroid hormone)(calcium).

6. An excess of thyroid hormone would cause (increased heart and respiratory rate and an increased appetite)(weight gain, hair loss, and fatigue).

7. Parathyroid hormone (PTH) activates (vitamin A)(vitamin D) to promote the absorption of calcium by the intestines.

Calcium balance is crucial to homeostasis. Review how the body achieves calcium balance by drawing arrows between the boxes to place the events in the proper sequence. (Note: There are two separate chains of events. One is for a blood calcium excess, and one is for a blood calcium deficiency.)

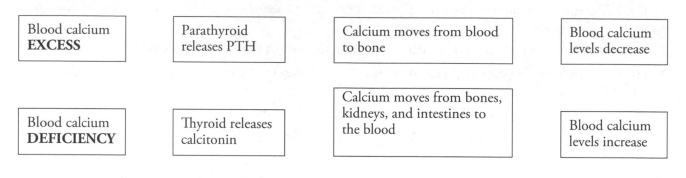

Blood calcium **EXCESS**	Parathyroid releases PTH	Calcium moves from blood to bone	Blood calcium levels decrease
Blood calcium **DEFICIENCY**	Thyroid releases calcitonin	Calcium moves from bones, kidneys, and intestines to the blood	Blood calcium levels increase

Drawing Conclusions: **Adrenal Glands**

Identify the two key structures of the adrenal cortex by coloring the adrenal medulla yellow and the adrenal cortex brown. Then complete the sentences to identify the actions of this endocrine gland. Circle the sentences related to the adrenal cortex in brown and those related to the adrenal medulla in yellow.

1. The adrenal medulla is part of the _____ nervous system; it secretes hormones called

   _____.

2. The adrenal cortex secretes hormones known as _____.

3. The adrenal cortex secretes a hormone that causes the kidneys to retain sodium (and excrete potassium), which leads to water retention. The name of this hormone is _____.

4. The adrenal cortex also secretes a hormone that helps the body adapt to stress and repair damaged tissue; the name of this hormone is _____.

Blood Glucose Regulation

The body must constantly work to keep blood glucose levels steady so as to provide cells with a steady supply of fuel. To improve your understanding of this process, fill in the blanks in the following sentences. Then enhance the figures next to each sentence by inserting arrows and hormone "dots" to illustrate what's occurring.

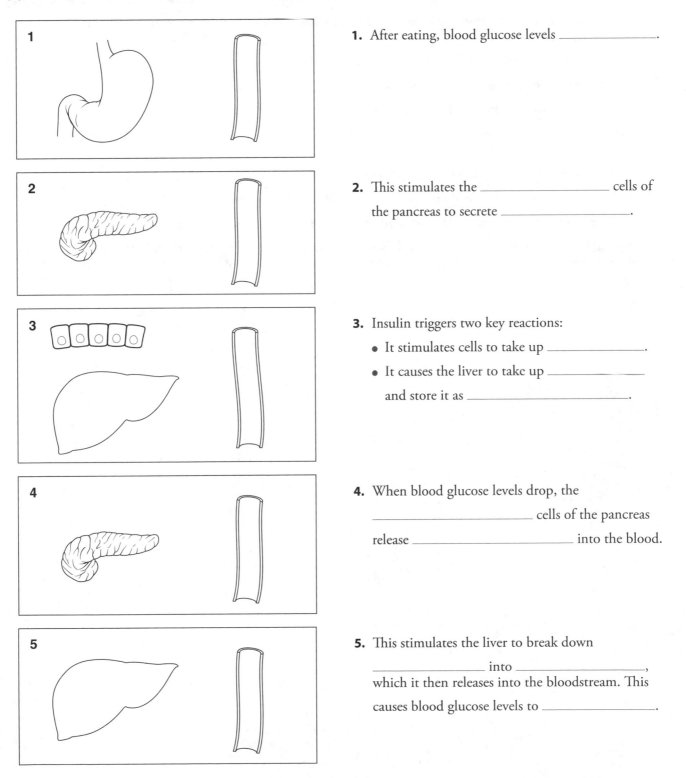

1. After eating, blood glucose levels _____.

2. This stimulates the _____ cells of the pancreas to secrete _____.

3. Insulin triggers two key reactions:
   - It stimulates cells to take up _____.
   - It causes the liver to take up _____ and store it as _____.

4. When blood glucose levels drop, the _____ cells of the pancreas release _____ into the blood.

5. This stimulates the liver to break down _____ into _____, which it then releases into the bloodstream. This causes blood glucose levels to _____.

Illuminate the Truth: Disorders of the Endocrine System

Use a highlighter to highlight the correct word or phrase in each sentence.

1. The secretion of too much growth hormone after epiphyseal plates have fused causes (gigantism)(acromegaly).

2. Low levels of (thyroid hormone)(melatonin) have been linked to mood disorders, particularly seasonal affective disorder.

3. Hypersecretion of thyroid hormone causes (simple goiter)(Graves' disease).

4. (Hypocalcemia)(Hypercalcemia) can lead to tetany.

5. Cushing syndrome results from (hyposecretion)(hypersecretion) of cortisol.

6. Hyposecretion of mineralocorticoids and glucocorticoids causes a disorder called (Addison's disease)(Graves' disease).

7. A lack of iodine results in (simple goiter)(hypoparathyroidism).

8. A diminished number of normal insulin receptors results in (hypoglycemia)(hyperglycemia).

9. In diabetes mellitus, the cells suffer from a(n) (insufficient)(surplus) amount of glucose.

10. If a child is born without a thyroid, he will develop a disorder called (dwarfism)(cretinism), which is characterized by retarded growth and sexual development, a low metabolic rate, and mental retardation.

More Endocrine Information

Further test your knowledge of the endocrine system by completing the following crossword puzzle.

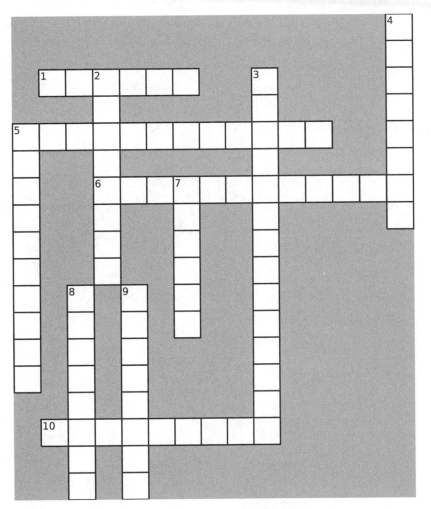

ACROSS

1. Primary sex organs
5. Hormone secreted by the corpus luteum after ovulation
6. Hormone that stimulates the development of secondary sexual characteristics in males
10. Antidiuretic hormone _____ urine volume.

DOWN

2. Hormone secretion is often controlled by _____ feedback.

3. Chemical messengers released within the tissues where they are produced
4. Hormone secreted by the cells of the ovarian follicle
5. Term for excessive thirst (often a symptom of diabetes)
7. Gland that helps in the development of the immune system
8. Endocrine gland containing cell clusters called the islets of Langerhans
9. Term for excessive urination (often a symptom of diabetes)

13
BLOOD

Blood is actually a connective tissue. Unique because of its fluid matrix, blood serves as the body's transport medium: It delivers oxygen and removes waste products from the body's cells; it transports nutrients, hormones, and enzymes; it helps protect the body against infection; and it helps stabilize body temperature. What's more, analyzing blood components gives clues about the body's state of health. Use the exercises in this chapter to improve your understanding of this vital fluid.

Illuminate the Truth: Red Blood Cells

Highlight the correct word or phrase to complete each sentence about red blood cells.

1. Immature red blood cells—as well as white blood cells and platelet-producing cells—arise from (pluripotent stem cells)(lymphatic tissue).

2. Red blood cells (have a fixed shape)(are flexible).

3. Red blood cells (have a large nucleus)(have no nucleus), which means they (cannot replicate)(replicate easily).

4. How much oxygen the blood can carry depends on the quantity of (plasma)(red blood cells).

5. Red blood cells affected by sickle cell disease are (overly flexible)(overly stiff), causing them to elongate when they enter narrow vessels.

6. Each red blood cell contains (millions of hemoglobin molecules)(a single molecule of hemoglobin).

7. Red blood cells have a life span of about (365 days)(120 days).

Fill in the following crossword puzzle to test your knowledge of some key terms related to the blood.

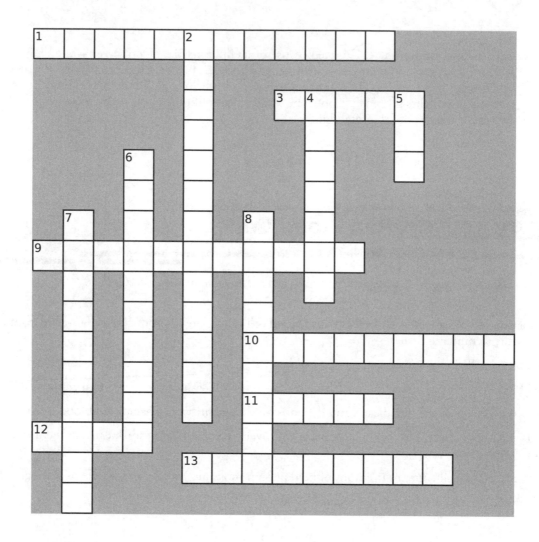

ACROSS

1. Blood contains more of this formed element than any other
3. Main component of plasma
9. Production of blood
10. White blood cell
11. Plasma without the clotting proteins
12. Necessary in the diet for hemoglobin synthesis
13. Property of blood determined by the combination of plasma and blood cells

DOWN

2. An increased number of these cells reflects an increase in the production of RBCs
4. The main protein in plasma
5. Most blood cells are created in _____ bone marrow
6. Red pigment that gives blood its color
7. Concentration of RBCs in a sample of blood
8. Excessive destruction of red blood cells

Hemoglobin

Over one-third of the interior of a red blood cell is filled with hemoglobin. Fill in the blanks in the following sentences to answer key questions about hemoglobin. Then color the figure as described.

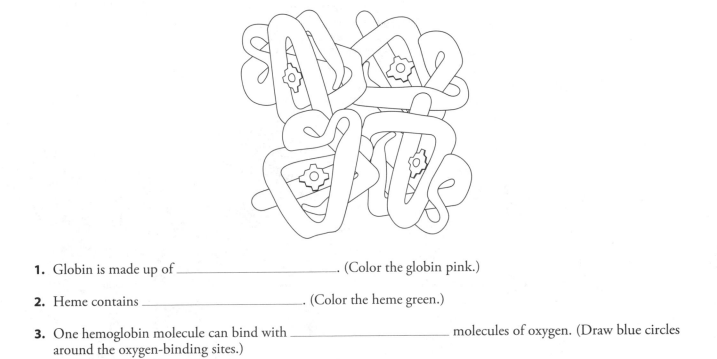

1. Globin is made up of _____. (Color the globin pink.)

2. Heme contains _____. (Color the heme green.)

3. One hemoglobin molecule can bind with _____ molecules of oxygen. (Draw blue circles around the oxygen-binding sites.)

4. When hemoglobin is saturated with oxygen, it is called _____.

Sequence of Events: **The Formation of Red Blood Cells**

The body must constantly produce new red blood cells to maintain homeostasis. Demonstrate your understanding of the life cycle of red blood cells by placing the following events in the proper sequence. For example, place a number 1 in the blank line before the first event in the sequence, a number 2 by the second event, and so on.

_____ **A.** An immature form of an erythrocyte, called a reticulocyte, is released into the circulation.

_____ **B.** EPO stimulates stem cells in red bone marrow to begin creating new erythrocytes.

_____ **C.** After one to two days, the reticulocyte becomes a mature erythrocyte.

_____ **D.** The kidneys detect the declining levels of oxygen and respond by secreting a hormone called erythropoietin (EPO).

_____ **E.** As the number of RBCs increases, oxygen levels rise. Less EPO is produced, and RBC production declines.

_____ **F.** As damaged RBCs are removed from circulation, oxygen levels fall.

The Breakdown of Red Blood Cells

Just as new red blood cells are continually formed, old blood cells are recycled. Describe this process, using the illustrations provided as clues. The first step in the process has been provided to get you started.

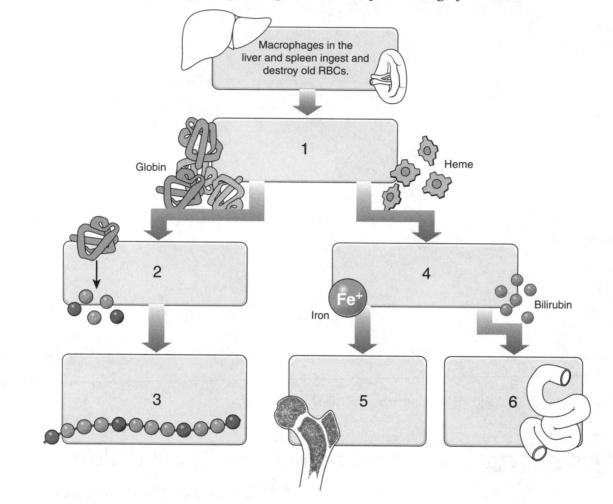

Macrophages in the liver and spleen ingest and destroy old RBCs.

Globin

Heme

1

2

4

Iron

Fe⁺

Bilirubin

3

5

6

1. _____
   _____

2. _____
   _____

3. _____
   _____

4. _____
   _____

5. _____
   _____

6. _____
   _____

Fill in the Gaps: Red Blood Cell Disorders

Fill in each of the blanks to correctly complete the following sentences about common blood disorders. Choose from the list of words in the Word Bank. (Hint: Not all the words will be used.)

ANEMIA	**JAUNDICE**	**POLYCYTHEMIA**	**SICKLE CELL ANEMIA**
HEMOLYTIC ANEMIA	**PERNICIOUS ANEMIA**	**PROTEINURIA**	**IRON DEFICIENCY ANEMIA**

1. The disease caused by an excess of RBCs is called _____.

2. A deficiency of RBCs is called _____.

3. A disorder that causes the excessive destruction of RBCs is _____.

4. A dietary deficiency of iron will cause _____.

5. A lack of vitamin B$_{12}$ causes _____.

6. A disorder common to African Americans that causes RBCs to elongate and clump together is called

   _____.

Just the Highlights: Granulocytes

Granulocytes—one of the two classifications of white blood cells—can be one of three types. Color each type of granulocyte a different color, such as the neutrophil yellow, the eosinophil blue, and the basophil green. Then link each cell to its characteristics by highlighting the sentences that describe neutrophils yellow, eosinophils blue, and basophils green.

Neutrophil Eosinophil Basophil

1. The fewest of the WBCs, making up 0.5% to 1% of the WBC count
2. Numerous in the lining of the respiratory and digestive tract
3. Most abundant of the WBCs, making up 60% to 70% of all the WBCs in circulation
4. Kill parasites
5. Account for 2% to 5% of circulating WBCs
6. Are sometimes called band cells or stab cells
7. Secrete heparin
8. Quickly move out of blood vessels into tissue spaces to engulf and digest foreign materials
9. Possess little to no phagocytic ability
10. Form the main component of pus
11. Involved in allergic reactions
12. Secrete histamine

Agranulocytes—the second classification of white blood cells—can be one of two types. Unscramble the words on the left to discover the names of those two types. Then draw a line to link each cell to its particular characteristics.

1. CLOTHEMYSPY

_ _ _ _ _ _ _ _ _ _ _ _

2. TYCOONSME

_ _ _ _ _ _ _ _ _ _

a. Are the smallest WBCs

b. Comprise 3% to 8% of the WBC count

c. Responsible for long-term immunity

d. May mature in the bone marrow or may migrate to the thymus to finish developing

e. Are largest WBCs

f. Are highly phagocytic; can engulf large bacteria as well as virus-infected cells

g. Colonize the organs and tissues of the lymph system when mature

h. May survive a few weeks to decades

i. Transform into macrophages in the tissues, where they ingest bacteria, cellular debris, and cancerous cells

j. May survive for several years

k. Are the second most numerous WBCs, making up 25% to 33% of the WBC count

Formation of a Blood Clot

Blood clotting involves a complex series of events. Test your knowledge of these events by placing the following reactions in the proper order. Place a number 1 in the blank by the first reaction, a 2 in the blank by the second reaction, and so on.

_____ **A.** Sticky fibrin threads form a web at the site of the injury.

_____ **B.** Both the intrinsic and extrinsic pathways result in the production of the enzyme prothrombin activator.

_____ **C.** Thrombin transforms the soluble plasma protein fibrinogen into insoluble fibrin.

_____ **D.** Red blood cells and platelets become ensnared in the fibrin web to create a clot of fibrin, blood cells, and platelets.

_____ **E.** Prothrombin is converted to the enzyme thrombin.

_____ **F.** Prothrombin activator acts on the globulin prothrombin (factor II).

List for Learning: # Preventing Clot Formation

List three factors that discourage blood clot formation.

1. _____

2. _____

3. _____

Blood Clotting

Complete the following crossword puzzle to strengthen your knowledge of key concepts in blood clotting.

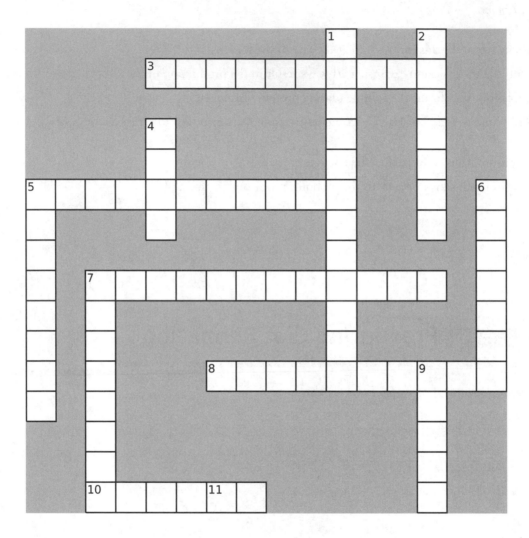

ACROSS

3. Rare disorder resulting from a deficiency of one of the clotting factors
5. Term for blood clotting
7. Another name for platelets
8. Stopping bleeding
10. A rough spot inside a blood vessel makes platelets become this

DOWN

1. Process of breaking up a blood clot
2. Adequate blood level of this mineral is required for clotting
4. A mass of platelets that forms a temporary seal on a vessel wall is called a platelet _____.
5. Fibers that are exposed when a vessel is injured
6. When a piece of a clot breaks off and circulates through the bloodstream
7. Unwanted blood clot inside a vessel
9. The first thing a blood vessel does when cut.
11. Vitamin necessary for clotting

Blood Types

Fill in the blanks to complete each of the following sentences. Choose from the words listed in the Word Bank.
(Hint: Not all the words will be used; also, words may be used more than once.)

AGGLUTINATION	**HEMOLYSIS**	**POSITIVE**	**B**
ANTIBODIES	**NEGATIVE**	**RED BLOOD CELLS**	**O**
ANTIGEN	**PLASMA**	**A**	**AB**

1. Each red blood cell carries a protein called an _____, of which there are two types (A and B).

2. Plasma carries _____ against the _____ of the other blood types.

3. A transfusion reaction occurs when the antibodies of one blood type attack the cells of the other blood type, causing the cells to clump together; the process of producing large clumps of cells is called _____.

4. During a reaction, red blood cells may burst; this is called _____.

5. Blood type _____ is sometimes called the universal donor, although the term is not completely accurate. Reactions usually don't occur because only the _____ are being transfused.

6. Blood type _____ is sometimes called the universal recipient, although this is not completely accurate either.

7. Many people also carry another antigen, called the Rh antigen; when this is the case, they are said to have Rh-_____ blood.

Improve your understanding of what happens when a woman with Rh-negative blood becomes pregnant with an Rh-positive fetus by doing the following:

- First, highlight the correct word or phrase in the sentences underneath each of the following illustrations.
- Next, illustrate what is occurring by inserting symbols for Rh-negative blood, Rh-positive blood, and anti-Rh antibodies. Use arrows to indicate the movement of the blood and antibodies. Finally, draw any reaction that may occur.

A. The first pregnancy of an Rh-negative mother with an Rh-positive fetus is (normal)(complicated).

B. During delivery, or miscarriage, the fetus' blood often (separates from)(mixes with) that of the mother, thus introducing (Rh antibodies)(Rh antigens) into the mother's bloodstream.

C. The mother's body responds by forming (anti-Rh antibodies)(Rh antigens).

D. If the mother becomes pregnant with another Rh-positive fetus, the (anti-Rh antibodies)(Rh antigens) in her body can pass through the placenta and attack the fetal RBCs, causing (hemophilia)(agglutination).

14
HEART

The structure of the heart allows it to serve as two distinct pumps. One side of the heart pumps blood to the lungs while the other side propels oxygenated blood throughout the body. The heart is unique in other ways as well. For example, it consists of muscle found nowhere else in the body. What's more, cardiac cells can generate and transmit electrical impulses spontaneously. Learn more about the characteristics of this vital organ by completing the activities in this chapter.

Conceptualize in Color: Heart Layers

Test your knowledge of the layers of the heart's wall and the pericardium by coloring the figure as suggested.

- Endocardium: Light pink
- Myocardium: Dark pink
- Fibrous pericardium: Orange

- Serous pericardium: Light blue
- Place green *X*s in the pericardial space.
- Draw a bracket linking the layers that make up the serous pericardium.

Complete the following crossword puzzle to test your knowledge of terms used in the study of the heart.

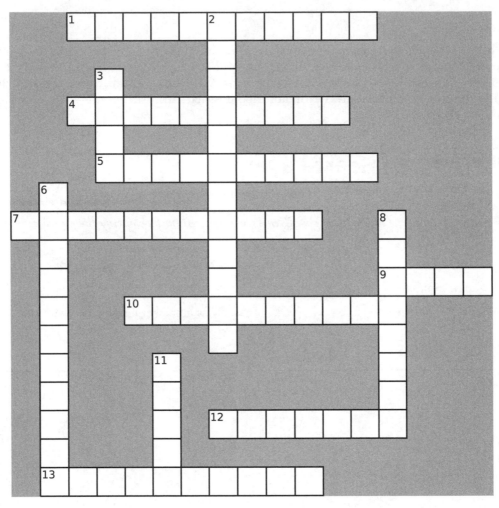

ACROSS

1. The heart's inner layer
4. The study of the heart and the treatment of related disorders
5. Thin layer of squamous epithelial cells covering the heart's surface
7. Space between the lungs and beneath the sternum where the heart resides
9. Pointed end of the heart
10. Two lower chambers of the heart
12. Phase of the cardiac cycle when the ventricles contract
13. Heart's middle layer

DOWN

2. Unique ability of the cardiac muscle to contract without nervous stimulation
3. Where the great vessels enter and leave the heart
6. Double-walled sac surrounding the heart and root of the great vessels
8. The period of cardiac muscle relaxation
11. Two upper chambers of the heart

Heart Structures

Color the heart structures in the following figure; use the colors suggested or choose your own. Then identify each of the heart's four valves (noted by the letters A through D in the figure) and describe the function of each; use the spaces provided.

- Right atrium: Dark blue
- Right ventricle: Light blue
- Left atrium: Light red
- Left ventricle: Dark red

- Interatrial septum: Orange
- Interventricular septum: Yellow
- Tendinous cords (chordae tendineae): Black
- Papillary muscle: Brown

Heart valves and functions:

A. _____

B. _____

C. _____

D. _____

Illuminate the Truth: Heart Valves

Highlight the correct word or phrase in each of the following sentences.

1. (Nerve impulses) (Pressure changes within the heart) trigger the opening and closing of the heart's valves.

2. A heart valve that fails to prevent the backflow of blood during contraction is called (incompetent) (stenotic), and the condition it causes is called valvular insufficiency.

3. (Valvular stenosis) (Regurgitation) is a condition resulting when a heart valve becomes narrowed, such as from scar tissue.

4. The mitral valve consists of (three) (two) cusps or leaflets.

5. The pulmonary and aortic valves are also called (semilunar) (tricuspid) valves.

6. The valves regulating flow between the atria and the ventricles are called (atrioventricular) (semilunar) valves.

7. The semi-rigid, fibrous connective tissue encircling each valve is called the (skeleton) (epicardium) of the heart.

8. Tendinous cords called chordae tendineae work to (pull the valves open when the heart contracts) (keep the tricuspid valve from inverting during ventricular contraction).

Drawing Conclusions: Heart Sounds

When heart valves close, they produce vibrations that can be heard with a stethoscope on the body's surface. In the following figure, identify the areas where each valve can be heard by coloring the circles as suggested; then fill in the name of each valve.

- Pulmonic area: Blue
- Mitral area: Yellow
- Tricuspid area: Green
- Aortic area: Orange

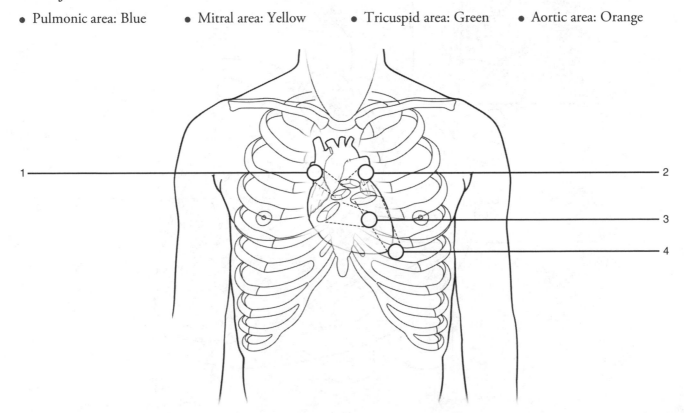

Sequence of Events: **Blood Flow Through the Heart**

Test your knowledge of the flow of blood through the heart by placing the following cardiac events in the proper order. The first step has been provided to get you started. Arrange the subsequent events by inserting the numbers 2 through 18 in the spaces provided.

1. Deoxygenated blood flows through the superior and inferior vena cava and into the right atrium.

_____ **A.** Blood fills the left atrium.

_____ **B.** The right atrium contracts.

_____ **C.** The pulmonary valve closes.

_____ **D.** Blood leaves the lungs via the pulmonary veins.

_____ **E.** The left atrium contracts.

_____ **F.** The pulmonary valve opens.

_____ **G.** Blood flows into the aorta for distribution throughout the body.

_____ **H.** The mitral valve closes.

_____ **I.** The left ventricle contracts.

_____ **J.** The aortic valve opens.

_____ **K.** The right ventricle contracts.

_____ **L.** The tricuspid valve opens.

_____ **M.** Blood is pumped into the right and left pulmonary arteries and into the lungs.

_____ **N.** Blood fills the left ventricle.

_____ **O.** The mitral valve opens.

_____ **P.** Blood flows into the right ventricle.

_____ **Q.** The tricuspid valve snaps closed.

Coronary Circulation

Fill in the blanks to complete the sentences. Choose from the words provided in the Word Bank. **(Hint:** *Not all the words will be used.)*

ANTERIOR DESCENDING	CORONARY SINUS	RELAXATION
ASCENDING AORTA	INTERVENTRICULAR SEPTUM	RIGHT
CIRCUMFLEX	LEFT	SUPERIOR VENA CAVA
CONTRACTION	LEFT VENTRICLE	

1. The right and left coronary arteries arise from the _____.

2. The _____ coronary artery supplies blood to the right atrium, part of the left atrium, most of the right ventricle, and the inferior part of the left ventricle.

3. The left coronary artery branches into the _____ and _____ arteries.

4. The left coronary artery supplies blood to the left atrium, most of the left ventricle, and most of the _____.

5. Most cardiac veins empty into the _____, a large transverse vein on the heart's posterior, which returns blood to the right atrium.

6. The coronary arteries receive their supply of blood during ventricular _____.

7. The most abundant blood supply goes to the myocardium of the _____.

Pacemakers of the Heart

List the heart's three possible pacemakers (the primary pacemaker as well as the "backup" pacemakers) along with their firing rates.

1. _____

2. _____

3. _____

In the following illustration, color and then label the structures of the cardiac conduction system. Use the colors suggested or choose your own.

- SA node: Red
- AV node: Green
- Bundle of His: Purple
- Right and left bundle branches: Blue

- Purkinje fibers: Pink
- Interatrial tracts: Brown
- Internodal tracts: Orange

Next, indicate the conduction pathway by placing a number by each of the labels, beginning by placing the number 1 by the name of the structure where the impulse begins and the number 7 by the structure where the impulse ends.

Color each part of the ECG waveform shown here as suggested.

- P wave: Green
- QRS complex: Yellow
- PR interval: Purple

- ST segment: Brown
- T wave: Blue

Next, link each part of the waveform to the cardiac activity it represents by underlining each particular statement with the color you used in the waveform. For example, if you colored the P wave green, underline in green the statement describing what the P wave represents.

1. This part of the waveform represents ventricular repolarization.

2. This part of the waveform represents atrial depolarization.

3. This part of the waveform represents the time it takes for the cardiac impulse to travel from the atria to the ventricles.

4. This part of the waveform represents ventricular depolarization.

5. This part of the waveform represents the end of ventricular depolarization and the beginning of ventricular repolarization.

The following illustrations show the five events of the cardiac cycle. Identify each event by filling in the blanks below each figure. Circle the name of the event when the first heart sound can be heard. Underline the name of the event when the second heart sound can be heard.

1   2   3   4   5

1. _____

2. _____

3. _____

4. _____

5. _____

Cardiac Output

*Place one word in each blank line to complete the following sentences. Choose from the words listed in the Word Bank. (**Hint:** Not all the words will be used; also, one word will be used more than once.)*

CARDIAC OUTPUT	**FIVE**	**PARASYMPATHETIC**	**SYMPATHETIC**
DECREASES	**HEART RATE**	**SIX**	**TEN**
EIGHT	**INCREASES**	**STROKE VOLUME**	

1. The amount of blood ejected with each heartbeat is called _____.

2. The amount of blood the heart pumps in 1 minute is called _____.

3. To determine cardiac output, you would multiply _____ by _____.

4. The average resting cardiac output is between _____ and _____ liters per minute.

5. When heart rate increases, cardiac output _____.

6. The nervous system can cause the heart rate to increase by sending impulses via the _____ nervous system.

7. The _____ nervous system sends signals to slow the heart rate.

Stroke Volume

Highlight the correct word in each of the following sentences.

1. (Preload)(Afterload) is the amount of tension, or stretch, in the ventricular muscle just before it contracts.

2. (Contractility)(Stroke volume) is the force with which ventricular ejection occurs.

3. Starling's law of the heart states that the more the ventricle is stretched—within limits—the (less)(more) forcefully it will contract.

4. The force against which the heart must work to eject its volume of blood is called the (cardiac output)(afterload).

5. Factors that affect contractility are called (chronotropic)(inotropic) agents.

6. Factors that affect heart rate are called (diastolic)(chronotropic) agents.

Make a Connection: Congestive Heart Failure

Unscramble the following words to discover the two types of heart failure. Then draw lines to link each type to its symptoms.

1. GIRTH CURRANTVEIL AREFLUI

   _ _ _ _ _   _ _ _ _ _ _ _ _ _ _ _

   _ _ _ _ _ _ _

2. FELT CAVALIERRUNT AIREFUL

   _ _ _ _   _ _ _ _ _ _ _ _ _ _ _

   _ _ _ _ _ _ _

a. Shortness of breath

b. Swelling of ankles, feet, and fingers

c. Enlargement of the liver and spleen

d. Pulmonary edema

e. Distention of jugular veins

f. Generalized swelling

g. Coughing

h. Pooling of fluid in the abdomen

Hone your knowledge of the heart by completing the following crossword puzzle.

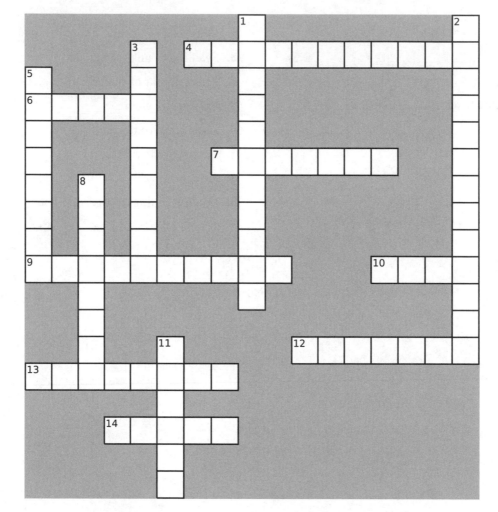

ACROSS

4. A persistent pulse rate slower than 60 beats per minute
6. An ECG that appears normal is called normal _____ rhythm.
7. Pacemakers other than the SA node are called this
9. An irregular heartbeat
10. The ventricle with the thickest walls
12. Pooling of fluid in the abdomen
13. The blood remaining in the ventricles at the end of the ejection period is the _____ volume.
14. The gender most likely to die from a first heart attack

DOWN

1. A persistent, resting heart rate greater than 100 beats per minute
2. Pressure sensors in the aorta and internal carotid arteries that detect changes in blood pressure
3. The right and left ventricles receive 70% of their blood _____.
5. Results from an interruption of blood to the myocardium
8. Cell death
11. Heart sound that results from turbulent blood flow through a stenotic valve

15
VASCULAR SYSTEM

The vascular system consists of an elaborate network of vessels designed to deliver oxygen and nutrients to the body's cells, remove waste products, and carry hormones from one part of the body to another. Varying in size and structure according to their purpose, many of these vessels have names that are important to remember. Use this chapter to learn the names of the various vessels and also to review their structure and function.

Drawing Conclusions: **Vessel Structure**

The walls of arteries and veins consist of three layers. Color and label each of these layers in the following figure. Then, in the corresponding space below the figure, identify the type of tissue making up each layer as well as the mechanism allowing the vessel to change diameter (if applicable).

1. _____

2. _____

3. _____

The body contains three types of arteries. Unscramble the following words to discover the names of these types. Then draw lines to link each artery to its characteristics.

1. DUCTCOGINN

— — — — — — — — — —

2. TIDBITSRUING

— — — — — — — — — — — —

3. EARLIESTOR

— — — — — — — — — —

a. These are the body's largest arteries.

b. Also called muscular arteries, these arteries have names.

c. These are the smallest arteries.

d. These are also called resistance vessels.

e. Also called elastic arteries, these arteries have names.

f. These vessels are too numerous to be named.

g. Examples include the aorta, common carotid, and subclavian arteries.

h. Examples include the brachial, femoral, and renal arteries.

i. These are connected to capillaries by short connecting vessels called metarterioles.

j. These arteries expand as blood surges into them and recoil when ventricles relax.

k. These arteries carry blood to specific organs and areas of the body.

Highlight in orange the sentences that pertain to large veins, the sentences that pertain to medium-sized veins in blue, and the sentences that pertain to venules in pink.

1. Contain one-way valves

2. Include the vena cavae, pulmonary veins, and internal jugular veins

3. Have a tunica media that is poorly developed, resulting in very thin vessel walls

4. Include the radial and ulnar veins of the forearm and the saphenous veins in the legs

5. Collect blood from the capillaries

6. Formed by the convergence of medium-sized veins

7. Formed by the convergence of venules on their route toward the heart

8. Are porous and can exchange fluid with surrounding tissue

Test your knowledge of vascular terms by completing the following crossword puzzle.

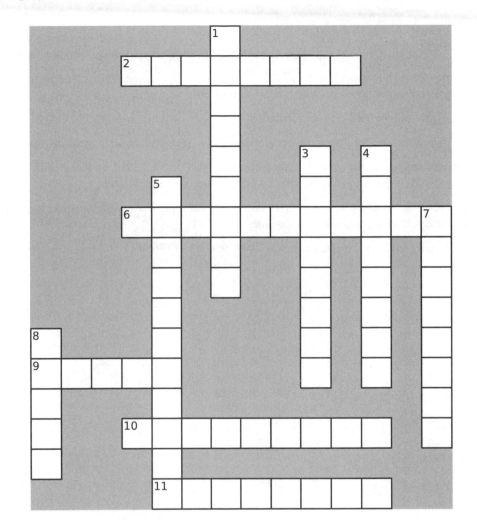

ACROSS

2. Results from the pressure of blood against a weakened area in the wall of an artery

6. Veins are sometimes called _____ vessels because of their capacity for storing blood.

9. Results when fluid filters out of the capillaries faster than it's reabsorbed and accumulates in the tissues

10. The most important mechanism of capillary exchange

11. The circulatory system that begins at the left ventricle and involves the circulation of blood through the body

DOWN

1. The circulatory system that begins at the right ventricle and involves the circulation of blood through the lungs

3. Vessels that carry blood away from the heart

4. Unique capillary found in liver and bone marrow that allows for passage of large substances, such as proteins

5. Where nutrients, wastes, and hormones are transferred between the blood and tissues

7. Capillaries are called the _____ vessels of the circulatory system.

8. Vessels that return blood to the heart

Chapter 15 Vascular System   *189*

Highlight the word or phrase that makes each of the following statements true.

1. Capillaries (are)(are not) evenly distributed throughout the body.

2. The majority of the capillaries in skeletal muscles are (constantly filled with blood)(shut down during periods of rest).

3. Capillaries (take up)(release) wastes, such as carbon dioxide and ammonia.

4. Water (flows into)(moves into and out of) capillaries.

5. In diffusion, substances move from areas of (greater)(lesser) to (greater)(lesser) concentration.

6. The concentration of oxygen within capillaries is (greater than)(less than) the concentration of oxygen in the surrounding tissue fluid; therefore, oxygen diffuses (into)(out of) the capillaries.

7. (Osmosis) (Filtration) occurs close to the arterial side of the capillary bed, while (colloid osmotic pressure)(diffusion) operates toward the venous side.

8. Of all the fluid filtered at the arterial end of the capillary bed, about (85%)(15%) is reabsorbed at the venous end.

Filtration and Osmotic Pressure

Fill in the blanks in the following sentences to correctly describe two methods of capillary exchange. As you proceed, use the space provided to illustrate the process described by each sentence. The first illustration and sentence are completed for you.

1. Blood enters the capillary through the metarteriole. The pressure here is about 30–35 mm Hg, while the pressure in the surrounding tissue fluid is about 2 mm Hg.

1

Tissue fluid pressure 2 mm Hg

Arterial blood

Pressure 30 mm HG

Arterial end

2. The higher pressure in the capillary pushes

_____ and _____

_____ through the capillary wall and

into the surrounding fluid. This is called _____

_____.

2

3. Meanwhile, as the blood moves toward the venous

end of the capillary, blood pressure inside the

capillary _____.

3

4. This allows the proteins in the blood, such as

albumin, to exert _____

_____, in which the albumin

in the blood pulls _____

_____ along with _____

into the capillaries.

4

List for Learning: Edema

List three main causes of edema.

1. _____

2. _____

3. _____

Sequence of Events: Pulmonary Circulation

Blood follows a specific route as it circulates through the lungs. Identify this path by placing the numbers 1 through 10 in the spaces provided. (Hint: Begin with the right ventricle.)

_____ **A.** Left atrium

_____ **B.** Venules

_____ **C.** Arterioles

_____ **D.** Lobar arteries in the lungs

_____ **E.** Pulmonary vein

_____ **F.** Veins

_____ **G.** Right ventricle

_____ **H.** Pulmonary arteries

_____ **I.** Lung capillaries

The Aorta

Color the regions of the aorta and its branches using the colors suggested, or choose your own colors.

- Ascending aorta: Blue
- Aortic arch: Green
- Descending aorta: Pink
- Abdominal aorta: Red
- Right common carotid: Orange

- Left common carotid: Orange
- Left subclavian artery: Purple
- Right subclavian artery: Purple
- Brachiocephalic artery: Brown
- Right and left common iliac arteries: Yellow

Color these principal arteries in the following figure using the colors suggested, or choose your own colors.

- Subclavian: Red
- Axillary: Green
- Brachial: Orange
- Radial: Purple
- Celiac trunk: Red
- Superior mesenteric: Blue
- Inferior mesenteric: Yellow
- Renal: Brown
- Common iliac: Pink
- Internal iliac: Green
- External iliac: Orange
- Femoral: Purple
- Popliteal: Green
- Anterior tibial: Blue
- Posterior tibial: Orange
- Dorsalis pedis: Red

Conceptualize in Color: Arteries of the Head and Neck

Identify and color the key arteries in the head and neck; use the colors suggested, or choose your own.

- Subclavian artery: Red
- Brachiocephalic: Orange
- Vertebral artery: Blue

- Common carotid: Yellow
- Internal carotid: Green
- External carotid: Purple

The Circle of Willis

Identify the circle of Willis in the figure by coloring these arteries. Use the colors suggested, or choose your own.

- Anterior cerebral arteries: Red
- Anterior communicating artery: Green
- Posterior communicating arteries: Orange
- Posterior cerebral arteries: Purple
- Basilar artery: Yellow
- Internal carotids: Dark blue

- Vertebral arteries: Brown
- Common carotid arteries: Pink
- Right and left subclavian arteries: Gray
- Brachiocephalic artery: Light blue
- Aortic arch: Dark red

Identify the principal veins in the following figure by coloring them as suggested, or choose your own colors.

- Basilic: Purple
- Cephalic: Orange
- Axillary: Pink
- Subclavian: Blue
- Brachiocephalic: Green
- Superior vena cava: Dark red
- Internal jugular: Orange
- External jugular: Purple
- Median cubital: Green
- Inferior vena cava: Tan
- External iliac: Red
- Internal iliac: Dark blue
- Common iliac: Yellow
- Hepatic: Light red
- Great saphenous: Brown
- Posterior tibial: Orange
- Anterior tibial: Gold
- Popliteal: Pink
- Femoral: Purple

Veins of the Head and Neck

Identify the key veins of the head and neck in the figure by coloring them as suggested, or choose your own colors.

- Internal jugular: Red
- Right subclavian: Yellow
- Brachiocephalic: Brown

- External jugular: Purple
- Vertebral: Green

Hepatic Portal Circulation

Identify the key veins of the hepatic portal circulation in the following figure by coloring them as suggested, or choose your own colors.

- Inferior vena cava: Red
- Hepatic veins: Orange
- Portal vein: Purple

- Superior mesenteric vein: Green
- Splenic vein: Yellow
- Inferior mesenteric vein: Pink

Circulation and Blood Pressure

Highlight the word or phrase to correctly complete each sentence.

1. A (portal)(venous) network is one in which blood flows through two sets of capillaries.

2. Blood always flows from an area of (higher)(lower) pressure to an area of (higher)(lower) pressure.

3. This difference in pressure is called a pressure (resistance)(gradient).

4. When the left ventricle contracts, it ejects blood into the aorta, producing a typical, normal blood pressure of (140 mm Hg)(110 mm Hg); this is called the (diastolic)(systolic) pressure.

5. When the ventricle relaxes, the pressure drops to an average of (70 mm Hg)(90 mm Hg); this is called the (diastolic)(systolic) pressure.

6. As blood moves away from the heart, blood pressure (remains constant)(continues to decline).

7. The greater the (pressure difference)(resistance) between two points, the greater the flow.

8. A lower than normal blood pressure is called (hypotension)(hypertension), while higher than normal blood pressure is called (hypotension)(hypertension).

9. A blood pressure of 128/84 mm Hg would be considered (normal)(prehypertension).

10. A blood pressure of 152/91 mm Hg would be considered (stage I hypertension)(stage II hypertension).

11. The opposition to flow resulting from the friction of moving blood against the vessel walls is called (high blood pressure)(peripheral resistance).

Maintenance of Blood Pressure

The maintenance of blood pressure is crucial for normal body functioning. The following chart lists three factors that determine blood pressure. In the spaces provided, describe how each factor influences blood pressure and provide formulas for each. Formulas for cardiac output have been provided to get you started.

	FACTOR	HOW FACTOR INFLUENCES BLOOD PRESSURE	FORMULA
1.	Cardiac output		$\uparrow CO = \uparrow BP$ $\downarrow CO = \downarrow BP$
2.	Blood volume		
3.	Resistance		

High and Low Blood Pressure

In the following list, highlight in yellow the factors that would cause blood pressure to rise; highlight in blue the factors that would cause a drop in blood pressure.

1. Increased blood viscosity

2. Vasodilation

3. Vasoconstriction

4. Hemorrhage

5. Atherosclerosis

6. Decreased number of red blood cells

7. Dehydration

8. Exercise

List for Learning: # Capillary Blood Flow

List four reasons why blood flow is slower in capillaries than in other parts of the vascular system.

1. _____

2. _____

3. _____

4. _____

Neural Regulation of Blood Pressure

The vascular system can quickly adjust blood pressure and alter the flow of blood to respond to the body's changing needs. Test your understanding of how the nervous system affects blood pressure by filling in the blanks in the following sentences. Choose from the words listed in the Word Bank.

AORTIC ARCH	**GLOSSOPHARYNGEAL**	**RISES**	**VASODILATION**
CAROTID SINUS	**MEDULLA**	**SYMPATHETIC**	**VAGUS**
DROPS	**PARASYMPATHETIC**	**VASOCONSTRICTION**	

1. Baroreceptors in the _____ and _____ detect changes in blood pressure and transmit signals along the _____ and _____ nerves to the cardiac control center and the vasomotor center in the _____.

2. If the pressure is too high:

   a. The medulla increases its output of _____ impulses.

   b. _____ occurs; heart rate and stroke volume decrease.

   c. Blood pressure _____.

3. If the blood pressure is too low:

   a. The medulla increases its output of _____ impulses.

   b. _____ occurs; heart rate and stroke volume increase.

   c. Blood pressure _____.

Hormonal Regulation of Blood Pressure

In the following list, highlight in pink the names of the hormone(s) that cause blood pressure to rise and highlight in blue the names of the hormone(s) that cause blood pressure to fall. (Hint: Not all the hormones listed will be highlighted.)

1. Epinephrine

2. Aldosterone

3. Insulin

4. Antidiuretic hormone (ADH)

5. Atrial natriuretic peptide (ANP)

6. Gastrin

7. Renin, angiotensin I, and angiotensin II

8. Norepinephrine

9. Estrogen

Describe the Process: Venous Return

Using the following illustrations as a guide, identify and describe the two key mechanisms that aid in venous return.

1. What mechanism is illustrated by the figure below? _____

How does this mechanism function? _____

_____

_____

_____

_____

_____

_____

2. What mechanism is illustrated by the figure below? _____

How does this mechanism function? _____

_____

_____

_____

_____

_____

_____

2

16
LYMPHATIC & IMMUNE SYSTEMS

The lymphatic and immune systems work together to protect the body against disease. The immune system consists primarily of a population of cells that defend the body against invasion by viruses, bacteria, and other disease-causing agents. These cells inhabit the lymphatic system: a network of organs and vessels that extend throughout the body.

Make a Connection: Lymphatic Organs

Patches of specialized tissue containing lymphocytes exist throughout the body. Lymphatic organs, however, are well defined. Unscramble the words on the left to discover the names of the lymphatic organs. Then draw lines to link each organ to its description or function. (Hint: Some organs have more than one correct answer.)

1. MYTHUS

— — — — — — —

2. MYPHL SNEDO

— — — — — — —   — — — — — —

3. LISTSNO

— — — — — — — —

4. PLESNE

— — — — — —

a. Consists of masses of lymphoid tissue that form a protective circle at the back of the throat

b. Analyzed to determine whether cancer has metastasized

c. The body's largest lymphatic organ

d. Large in children, this organ shrinks to a fraction of its former size by adulthood.

e. Besides cleansing lymph, also serve as sites for final maturation of some types of lymphocytes and monocytes

f. Provides a location for B and T lymphocytes to mature

g. Prone to injury, rupture of this organ could result in a fatal hemorrhage

h. Removes 99% of the impurities in lymph before it returns the fluid to the bloodstream

List for Learning: Functions of Lymph

Lymphatic vessels are filled with lymph: a clear, colorless fluid that originates in the tissues as the fluid left behind following capillary exchange. Using the spaces provided, list the three functions of lymph.

1. _____

2. _____

3. _____

Drawing Conclusions: Lymphatic Vessels

Although lymphatic vessels are similar to veins, they have some key differences. Review your knowledge of lymphatic vessels by first filling in the blanks with the correct word or words. Then follow the instructions after each sentence to color the figure as described.

1. Lymphatic vessels originate in _____ as microscopic, blind-ended

    sacs within a bed of _____.
    (*Color the lymphatic vessel shown in the figure green.*)

2. _____ flows into lymphatic vessels through gaps between cells. _____,

    _____, and _____ flow in with the fluid.
    (*Insert arrows in the figure to illustrate how fluid enters the vessel.*)

3. Valves prevent backflow, ensuring that lymph moves _____ from tissues and

    _____ the heart.
    (*Color the valves in the figure dark blue; insert arrows to show the direction of flow.*)

4. _____ anchor the lymphatic vessels to surrounding cells, which helps to

    keep the vessels from collapsing.
    (*Color these structures in the figure purple.*)

Overview of the Lymphatic System

The lymphatic system consists of lymphatic vessels, lymph, lymphatic tissue, and lymphatic organs. Identify the structures of the lymphatic system by coloring them as suggested or choose your own colors.

- Spleen: Red
- Red bone marrow: Pink
- Cervical lymph nodes: Green
- Axillary lymph nodes: Purple
- Inguinal lymph nodes: Orange
- Tonsils: Brown
- Thymus gland: Tan
- Trace the lymphatic vessels in blue
- Shade the area drained by the right lymphatic duct yellow
- Shade the area drained by the thoracic duct light purple

Lymph Node

As lymph flows through lymphatic vessels, it passes through multiple lymph nodes. Identify the structures of the lymph node using the colors suggested or choose your own colors.

- Fibrous capsule: Tan
- Trabeculae: Green
- Sinuses: Light blue

- Cortical nodules: Purple
- Germinal centers: Pink
- Afferent vessels: Brown

- Efferent vessel: Orange
- Insert arrows showing direction of lymph flow

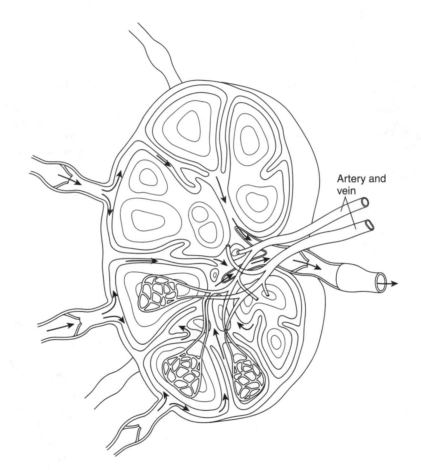

Artery and vein

Functions of the Spleen

The spleen is the body's largest lymphatic organ. Using the spaces provided, list four functions of this major lymphatic organ.

1. _____

2. _____

3. _____

4. _____

Build your knowledge about the spleen by filling in the blanks in the sentences with the correct word or words. Then color the splenic structures using the colors suggested or choose your own colors.

1. The spleen lies in the upper _____ quadrant of the abdomen.

2. The spleen is structurally similar to the _____.

3. Lymphocytes and macrophages in the _____ pulp screen the passing blood for foreign antigens.

4. Macrophages in the _____ remove and digest worn-out blood cells.

5. The spleen stores 20% to 30% of the body's _____.

6. The spleen produces _____ in the fetus.

Color the following structures:

- Spleen: Brown
- Venous sinuses: Purple
- White pulp: Yellow

- Red pulp: Pink
- Capsule: Tan
- Artery: Red

- Veins: Blue
- Splenic artery: Red
- Splenic vein: Blue

The Lymphatic System

Complete the crossword puzzle to review some key facts about the lymphatic system.

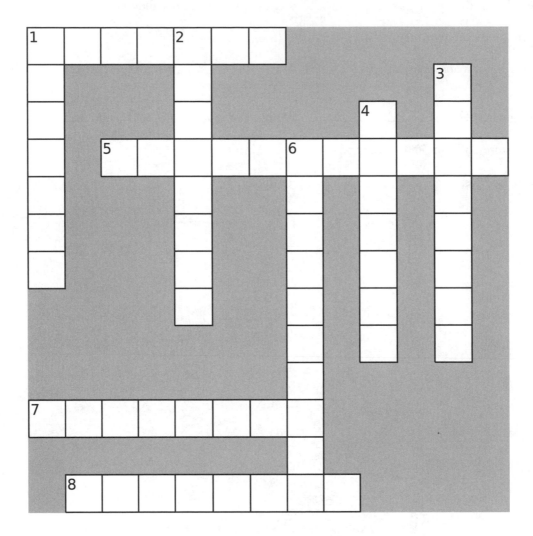

ACROSS

1. Red bone marrow and the thymus are known as _____ lymphatic organs because they provide a location for B and T lymphocytes to mature.
5. An acute inflammation of the tonsils
7. The tonsils most likely to become infected
8. Location of lymph nodes that monitor lymph coming from the head and neck

DOWN

1. Lymph has a lower _____ content than does plasma.
2. Term for pharyngeal tonsils
3. Lymph nodes through which most breast cancers metastasize
4. Tonsils concentrated in patches on either side of the tongue
6. Swelling that results when the lymphatic vessel is obstructed

Nonspecific Immunity

Nonspecific immunity uses a variety of mechanisms to protect the body against a broad range of pathogens. In the spaces provided, list six mechanisms of nonspecific immunity.

1. _____
2. _____
3. _____
4. _____
5. _____
6. _____

Drawing Conclusions: # Phagocytosis

Phagocytes are cells whose sole job is to ingest and destroy microorganisms. Review the process of phagocytosis by filling in the blanks in the sentences. Then follow the instructions to illustrate the process in the space provided.

1. The most important phagocytes are _____ and _____. When a

   phagocyte encounters a microorganism, it sends out membrane projections called _____.
   (In the space below, draw a cell sending out projections as described. Be sure to include a nucleus and lysosomes inside the cell. Also draw structures symbolizing bacteria outside the cell.)

2. The _____ envelops the organism, forming a complete sac called a _____.
(*Draw the second step in phagocytosis as described in sentence 2. Be sure to include a bacterium inside the second cell.*)

3. The _____ travels to the interior of the cell and fuses with a _____.
(*Draw a third cell showing the process of phagocytosis; illustrate what is being described in sentence number 3.*)

4. _____ from the _____ destroy the microorganism.
(Draw the final step in phagocytosis as described.)

Illuminate the Truth: **Process of Inflammation**

Tissue injury produces inflammation, which stimulates the immune system. Review the process of inflammation by highlighting the correct word or phrase in the following sentences.

1. Injured cells secrete chemicals, such as (histamine)(complement) that (constrict)(dilate) blood vessels in the area. Blood rushes in, bringing necessary (platelets)(leukocytes) and flushing out toxins and wastes.

2. The same chemicals cause the cells in the capillary walls to (constrict)(separate) slightly. Fluid, leukocytes, and plasma proteins—as well as antibodies, clotting factors, and complement—(flow into the capillary)(leak into the tissue).

3. (Neutrophils)(Platelets), which have been drawn to the area by chemicals released from damaged cells, (form a clot)(phagocytize the pathogens).

Review some of the aspects of the immune system by completing the following crossword puzzle.

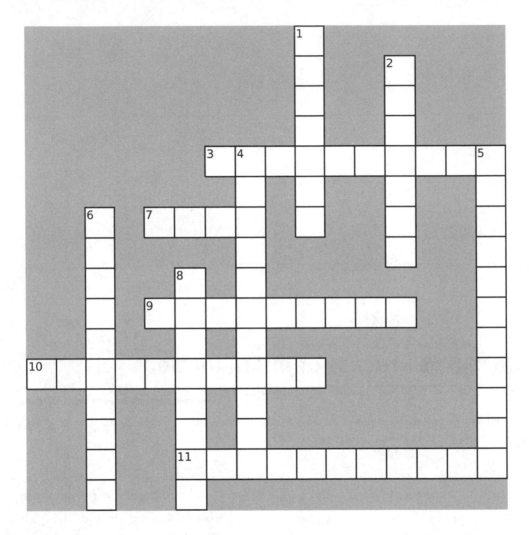

ACROSS

3. Antimicrobial protein secreted by a virus-infected cell
7. First line of defense against microorganisms
9. Area of increased blood flow
10. Immunoglobulins
11. Phagocytic white blood cells that congregate in areas where invasion is likely to occur

DOWN

1. An accumulation of pus within a cavity
2. Fever
4. Type of immunity aimed at a broad range of attackers
5. Phagocytic white blood cells that roam the body, seeking bacteria
6. Process whereby neutrophils are attracted to sites of infection as a result of a chemical released from inflamed cells
8. Enzyme found in mucus, tears, and saliva that destroys bacteria

Proteins called complement circulate in the bloodstream in inactive form. Once activated, a complement reaction begins. Test your understanding of this process by first filling in the blanks in each of the following sentences. Then follow the instructions to draw the process in the space provided.

1. _____ or _____ activate complement, triggering a cascade of

   chemical reactions. The final group of proteins, called the _____

   _____   _____, embed themselves into the bacterium's

   membrane in ring-like circles.
   (*On the left-hand side of the space below, draw a large oval to symbolize a bacterium. Draw small triangles outside the bacterium to symbolize complement. Draw the complement embedding in the wall of the bacterium in ring-like circles.*)

2. _____ and _____ rush into the bacterium through the openings.
   (*Draw another bacterium with the ring-like circles of complement embedded in the wall. Draw arrows and symbols to represent the process being described in sentence number 2.*)

3. The bacterium _____ and _____.
   (*Draw what is being described in sentence number 3.*)

Inflammation

List the four classic signs of inflammation.

1. _____

2. _____

3. _____

4. _____

Sequence of Events: **Fever**

Insert the numbers 1 through 7 in the spaces provided to place the events that occur during a fever in their proper order.

_____ **A.** The temperature rises until it reaches its new set point, where it remains as long as the pathogen is present.

_____ **B.** Neutrophils and macrophages secrete a fever-producing substance called a pyrogen.

_____ **C.** When the pathogen is no longer a threat, the phagocytes stop producing the pyrogen, and the body's set point for temperature returns to normal.

_____ **D.** The body loses excess heat through sweating and dilating the blood vessels in the skin, resulting in warm, flushed skin.

_____ **E.** PGE resets the body's set point for temperature.

_____ **F.** The body shivers and constricts the blood vessels in the skin, resulting in chills and cold, clammy skin.

_____ **G.** The pyrogen stimulates the anterior hypothalamus to secrete prostaglandin E (PGE).

Make a Connection: Classes of Immunity

Unscramble the words on the left to discover the four classes of immunity. Then draw lines to link each class of immunity with its characteristics.

1. ULTRAAN TEICAV

   _ _ _ _ _ _ _
   _ _ _ _ _ _

2. ACILIARIFT VATICE

   _ _ _ _ _ _ _ _ _ _
   _ _ _ _ _ _

3. LAATURN VASESPI

   _ _ _ _ _ _ _
   _ _ _ _ _ _ _

4. ITALICFARI PAVESIS

   _ _ _ _ _ _ _ _ _
   _ _ _ _ _ _ _

a. Results following an injection of serum from a person or animal that has produced antibodies against a pathogen

b. Occurs when the body produces antibodies or T cells after being exposed to a particular antigen

c. Follows a tetanus shot

d. Follows an infection with measles

e. Occurs through breastfeeding

f. Results when the body makes T cells and antibodies following a vaccination

g. Follows an injection for rabies

h. Results when a fetus acquires antibodies from the mother through the placenta

Illuminate the Truth: Specific Immunity

Review some of the key concepts about specific immunity by highlighting the correct word or phrase in each sentence.

1. (Cellular immunity)(Humoral immunity) destroys foreign cells or host cells that have become infected with a pathogen.

2. B cells mature in the (thymus)(bone marrow) while T cells mature in the (thymus)(bone marrow).

3. Also known as immunoglobulins, (antibodies)(antigens) are formed by B cells.

4. An (antigen)(allergen) is any molecule that triggers an immune response.

5. A secondary immune response (takes longer)(happens more quickly) than the primary immune response.

Cellular Immunity

Cellular immunity destroys pathogens that exist within a cell. Review key facts about cellular immunity by filling in the blanks to complete the following sentences. Choose from the words listed in the Word Bank. (Hint: Not all the words will be used; also, words may be used more than once.)

ANTIGEN PRESENTATION	**EFFECTOR CELLS**	**MEMORY T**
ANTIGEN-PRESENTING CELL (APC)	**HELPER T**	**PHAGOCYTE**
B	**INTERLEUKINS**	**T**
COMPLEMENT	**LEUKOCYTE**	**T CELL**
CYTOTOXIC T		

1. The immune process begins when a _____ ingests an antigen.

2. Called an _____, this cell displays fragments of the antigen on its surface—a process called _____, which alerts the immune system to the presence of a foreign antigen. When a _____ spots the foreign antigen, it binds to it.

3. This activates (or sensitizes) the _____, which begins dividing repeatedly to form clones. Some of these cells become _____ (such as _____ cells and _____ cells), which will carry out the attack, while others become _____ cells.

4. The _____ cell binds to the surface of the antigen and delivers a toxic dose of chemicals that will kill it.

5. _____ cells support the attack by secreting the chemical _____, which attracts neutrophils, natural killer cells, and macrophages. It also stimulates the production of

_____ and _____ cells.

Humoral Immunity

In contrast to cellular immunity, humoral immunity focuses on pathogens outside the cell. Review the process of humoral immunity by filling in the blanks in the following sentences. Choose from the words in the Word Bank. (Hint: Not all the words will be used. Also, words may be used more than once.)

ANTIBODIES	**EFFECTOR B**	**MEMORY B**
ANTIGENS	**HELPER T**	**PLASMA**
B CELL	**INTERLEUKINS**	**T CELL**

1. The surface of a _____ contains thousands of receptors for a specific antigen. When the antigen specific to that receptor comes along, it binds to the _____.

2. The _____ then engulfs the antigen, digests it, and displays some of the antigen's fragments on its surface. A _____ cell binds to the presented antigen and secretes _____, which activates the _____.

3. The _____ begins to rapidly reproduce, creating a clone, or family, of identical cells that are programmed against the same antigen.

4. Some of these cloned cells become _____ cells or _____ cells; most, though, become _____ cells.

5. The _____ cells secrete large numbers of _____.

Hypersensitivity

Highlight the correct word or phrase in each sentence.

1. When someone with a genetic disposition to an allergy is first exposed to the (allergen)(antigen), the body produces large amounts of the (antibody)(antigen) (IgE)(IgG).

2. This reaction (does)(does not) produce an allergic reaction, and the body is now (sensitized)(immune) to the offending substance.

3. When the person encounters the same substance or material at a later date, the (allergen)(antigen) binds to the (antibodies)(antigens) already in the body.

4. (B cells)(Mast cells) release (interleukins)(histamine) and other inflammatory chemicals that produce the symptoms of an allergy, such as runny nose, watery eyes, congestion, and hives.

17

RESPIRATORY SYSTEM

The respiratory and cardiovascular systems work closely together to provide the body with essential oxygen and to remove carbon dioxide. What's more, the respiratory system also influences your ability to speak, smell, and taste. Use this chapter to review the structures and function of the respiratory system.

List for Learning: Upper and Lower Respiratory Tract

List the structures of the upper and lower respiratory tracts.
Upper respiratory tract:

1. _____

2. _____

3. _____

4. _____

5. _____

Lower respiratory tract:

1. _____

2. _____

3. _____

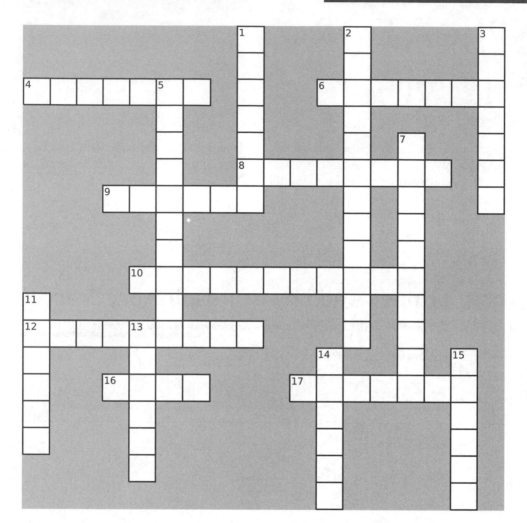

ACROSS

4. Portion of the respiratory tract that carries air through the neck and upper chest
6. Area of the brain that contains the centers for controlling breathing
8. Primary structure for gas exchange
9. Bony structure that separates the mouth from the nasal cavity
10. Type of pressure that drives respiration
12. During times of forced breathing, these muscles join in to aid respiratory effort.
16. The top of the lung
17. The opening between the vocal cords

DOWN

1. Three bones projecting from the lateral wall of the nasal cavity
2. A collapsed lung
3. Another name for throat
5. Closes over the top of the larynx during swallowing to direct food and liquids into the esophagus
7. Lipoprotein secreted by alveolar cells that decreases surface tension of the fluid lining the alveoli, permitting expansion
11. Respiratory structure where sound is produced
13. Vertical plate of bone and cartilage that separates the nasal cavity into two halves
14. Serous membrane covering the lungs and the thoracic cavity
15. Most common chronic illness in children

Conceptualize in Color: Nasal Cavity

Test your knowledge of the structures of the nasal cavity by coloring the following structures in the figure below:

- Nasal conchae: Pink
- Hard palate: Red
- Soft palate: Yellow

- Frontal sinus: Orange
- Sphenoid sinus: Blue
- Olfactory receptors: Green

Make a Connection: The Pharynx

Unscramble the following words to discover the names of the three regions of the pharynx. Then draw a line to link each region with its particular characteristics.

1. ANAXHORNSPY

— — — — — — — — — — — —

2. HARRYNOPOX

— — — — — — — — — — —

3. GRAYORPHANLYNX

— — — — — — — — — — — — — —

a. Space between the soft palate and the base of the tongue

b. Contains openings for the right and left auditory (Eustachian) tubes

c. Lies just behind the soft palate

d. Ends at the inferior end of the larynx (the beginning of the esophagus)

e. Contains the palatine and lingual tonsils

Highlight the correct word or words in each of the following sentences.

1. The larynx prevents (food and liquids)(dust) from entering the trachea.

2. The larynx acts as a passageway for (food)(air) between the pharynx and trachea.

3. The (vestibular folds)(vocal cords) found in the larynx produce sound.

4. The larynx is formed by nine (bones)(pieces of cartilage) that keep it from collapsing.

5. The opening between the vocal cords is called the (glottis)(epiglottis).

6. The vestibular folds, or false vocal cords, function to (close the glottis during swallowing)(form high-pitched sounds).

7. The "Adam's apple" is actually (the anterior portion of the trachea)(a large piece of cartilage called the thyroid cartilage).

The Larynx and Bronchial Tree

Color the structures of the larynx and bronchial tree in the following figure; use the suggested colors or choose your own.

- Larynx: Blue
- Trachea: Green
- Carina: Orange
- Primary bronchi: Yellow

- Secondary bronchus: Purple
- Tertiary bronchi: Pink
- Bronchioles: Tan

Fill in the Gaps: Alveoli

Fill in the blanks to correctly complete the following sentences. Choose from the words listed in the Word Bank. (Hint: Not all the words will be used.)

BLOOD	**CAPILLARIES**	**LIQUID**	**MEMBRANE**	**MUCUS**	**SURFACTANT**	**VEINS**

1. The alveoli are wrapped in a fine mesh of _____.

2. Gas exchange occurs through the respiratory _____.

3. For gas to enter or leave a cell, it must be dissolved in _____.

4. _____ is a substance that helps reduce surface tension inside the alveolus to keep it from collapsing.

Drawing Conclusions: The Lungs

Fissures divide the lungs into lobes. In the following figure, draw lines to show the locations of the fissures. Write the name of each fissure by the appropriate line. Then write the name of each lobe within the appropriate space inside the lungs.

In the following illustration, color the structures as suggested. Then, in the spaces provided, state the two purposes of pleural fluid.

- Visceral pleura: Green
- Parietal pleura: Orange
- Pleural space: Light blue

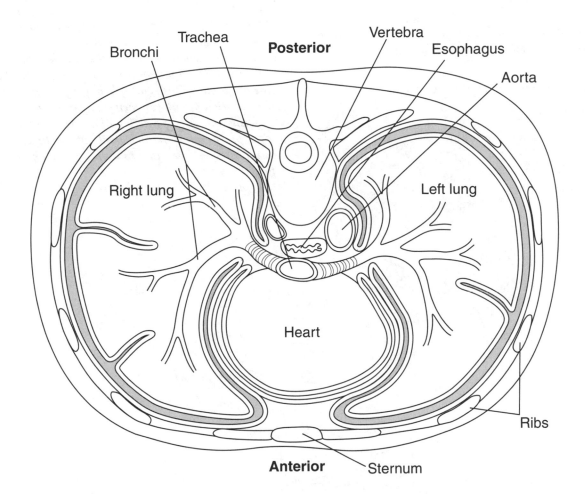

Pleural fluid serves two purposes:

1. _____

_____

2. _____

_____

Respiratory Muscles

Identify the muscles used for inspiration and expiration in the figure below by coloring them as suggested:

- External intercostal muscles: Pink
- Internal intercostal muscles: Green
- Diaphragm: Yellow

Identify the accessory muscles used for deep inspiration by coloring the following muscles as suggested:

- Sternocleidomastoids: Orange
- Scalenes: Purple
- Pectoralis minor: Light blue

Identify the accessory muscles used during forced expiration by coloring these muscles as suggested:

- Rectus abdominis: Brown
- External abdominal obliques: Gray

Next, identify the action of the muscles during inspiration. Use a black pen to insert arrows on the right side of the chest (the left side of the figure), showing the direction of pull for each group of muscles used.

Then identify the action of the muscles during expiration. Use a blue pen to insert arrows on the left side of the chest (the right side of the figure), showing the direction of pull for each group of muscles used.

Lastly, identify the action of accessory muscles. Use a red pen to insert arrows, showing the direction of pull for the muscles used in deep inspiration and forced expiration.

Neural Control of Breathing

Highlight the word or words that correctly completes each of the following sentences.

1. The skeletal muscles used for breathing (contract spontaneously)(require neural input to contract)

2. The centers for controlling breathing in the medulla (are interconnected)(operate independently).

3. The inspiratory center sends impulses to the intercostal muscles via the (vagus)(intercostal) nerves and to the diaphragm via the (phrenic)(glossopharyngeal) nerve to cause muscle contraction.

4. Exhalation results when (the expiratory center sends impulses to cause muscle relaxation)(nerve output ceases and the inspiratory muscles relax).

5. In the pons, the (apneustic)(pneumotaxic) center stimulates the inspiratory center to increase the length and depth of inspiration.

6. Also in the pons, the (apneustic)(pneumotaxic) center helps prevent overinflation of the lungs.

7. The (medulla)(cerebral cortex) allows for voluntary control of breath for activities such as singing.

8. (Oxygen)(Carbon dioxide) levels are the primary regulator of respiration.

Describe the Process: Factors Influencing Breathing

The respiratory center can alter breathing patterns in response to a number of factors. (Five such factors are shown in a table in the textbook entitled "Factors Influencing Breathing.") In the table below, identify the sensory receptor for each factor by filling in the blanks. Then describe what happens when each of these sensory receptors is activated, using the spaces provided. Some information has been provided to get you started.

FACTOR	SENSORY RECEPTOR	ACTION
Oxygen	_____ chemoreceptors (located in the _____ and _____ bodies)	Low blood levels of oxygen cause: As a result:

Continued

FACTOR	SENSORY RECEPTOR	ACTION
Hydrogen ions (pH)	_____ chemoreceptors (located in the _____ _____)	Declining pH levels indicate: When pH falls, these chemoreceptors signal the respiratory centers to:
Stretch	Receptors in the _____ and _____	Receptors detect stretching during inspiration and: This is called the:
Pain and emotion	_____ and _____ system	In response to pain and emotion:
Irritants (such as smoke, dust, pollen, noxious chemicals, and mucus)	_____ in the airway	These receptors respond to irritants by: This helps to:

Illuminate the Truth: Pressure and Airflow

Highlight the correct words or phrases in each of the following sentences.

1. Air moves in and out of lungs because of a (pressure)(oxygen) gradient.

2. When the pressure within the lungs drops lower than atmospheric pressure, (inspiration)(expiration) occurs; when it rises above atmospheric pressure, (inspiration)(expiration) occurs.

3. The thin film of fluid between the visceral and parietal pleura (causes them to cling together)(keeps them separated), aiding lung expansion.

4. The potential space between the two pleura maintains a pressure slightly (less)(greater) than atmospheric pressure; this is called (negative)(positive) pressure.

The Respiratory Cycle

Review the process of inspiration and expiration in two ways. First, insert the correct word or phrase in the blanks in each sentence. Then illustrate the process by inserting arrows into the figure as described.

Inspiration:

1. The intercostal muscles _____, pulling the ribs up and out; the diaphragm contracts and moves _____. (*Insert red arrows in the drawing above to illustrate this part of the process.*)

2. The lungs _____ along with the chest. (*Insert green arrows to illustrate what's happening.*)

3. The pressure within the bronchi and alveoli _____. (*Insert a black arrow inside the lung next to a letter P to indicate the change in pressure.*)

4. When intrapulmonic pressure _____ than atmospheric pressure, air flows _____ the lungs. (*Insert blue arrows to indicate the direction of air flow.*)

Expiration:

1. The diaphragm and external intercostals _____ and the thoracic cage
_____ to its original size. *(Insert red arrows in the drawing above to illustrate this part of the process.)*

2. The lungs are _____ by the thoracic cage. *(Insert green arrows to illustrate what is happening.)*

3. Intrapulmonary pressure _____. *(Insert a black arrow inside the lung next to a letter P to indicate the change in pressure.)*

4. Air flows _____ of the lungs. *(Insert blue arrows to indicate the direction of air flow.)*

Fill in the blanks to complete the following sentences about measuring lung capacity. Then follow the instructions to create a spirographic record. Use a pencil to create the waveform so that you can alter it as needed to complete each step.

1. The amount of air inhaled and exhaled during quiet breathing is known as _____. In a

   healthy young adult, this measurement is typically _____ mL.
   (Create a spirographic record in the rectangle below. Begin by inserting a waveform showing the measurement described in sentence 1. Use the numbers along the left of the rectangle as a guide. Color the area on the spirographic record indicative of this measurement blue. In other words, highlight the area behind the waveform blue. Write the name of the measurement in the blue area.)

2. The amount of air inhaled using maximum effort after a normal inspiration is called the _____

   _____ volume. This amount is typically _____ mL.
   (Alter the waveform to include this reading. Color the area on the spirographic record indicative of this measurement green; write the name of the measurement in the green area.)

3. The amount of air that can be exhaled after a normal expiration using maximum effort is the _____

   _____ volume. This amount is typically _____ mL.
   (Alter the waveform to include this reading. Color the area on the spirographic record indicative of this measurement orange and write the name of the measurement in the orange area.)

4. The amount of air remaining in the lungs after a forced expiration is called the _____

   _____. This amount is about _____ mL.
   (Color the area on the spirographic record indicative of this measurement pink; write the name of the measurement in this pink area.)

5. The amount of air that can be inhaled and exhaled with the deepest possible breath is the _____

   _____. This number can be obtained by adding the tidal volume to the

   _____ and _____ volumes.
   (Draw a bracket around the part or parts of the waveform that indicates this measurement. Label the bracket with the name of the measurement.)

6. The maximum amount of air that the lungs can contain is called the _____.
   (Draw a second bracket around the part or parts of the waveform that indicate this measurement. Label the bracket with the name of the measurement.)

Gas Exchange

Fill in the blanks to complete the following sentences about gas exchange in the alveoli. Then follow the instructions to illustrate the process.

1. Gas diffuses from an area of _____ pressure to _____ pressure until the pressures are equalized.

2. Air flowing into the alveoli has a partial pressure of oxygen that is _____ than the partial pressure of oxygen in the pulmonary capillaries.
   (In the following figure, insert the symbol for oxygen within the alveoli with an arrow showing whether the level of oxygen is high or low.)

3. The pulmonary capillaries surrounding the alveoli contain venous blood that contains a partial pressure of

   carbon dioxide that is _____ than the partial pressure of carbon dioxide in the alveoli.
   (Near the capillary, insert the symbol for carbon dioxide with an arrow showing whether the level is high or low.)

4. These differences in partial pressures cause oxygen to flow _____ the alveoli and

   _____ the capillaries.
   (Between the capillary and the alveoli, illustrate the direction of gas exchange by inserting red arrows to signify the movement of oxygen.)

5. Simultaneously, carbon dioxide flows _____ the alveoli and _____ the capillaries.
   (Insert blue arrows to show the movement of carbon dioxide across the capillary membrane. Next, color the blood cells with low levels of oxygen blue, color those with high levels of oxygen red, and those undergoing gas exchange purple.)

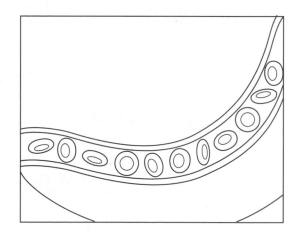

Gas Transport

Complete the following crossword puzzle to test your knowledge of gas transport. Also included are some terms used to describe variations in breathing.

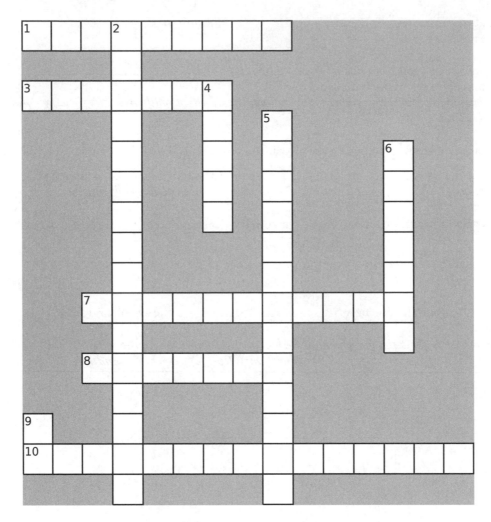

ACROSS

1. Labored breathing that occurs when a person is lying flat but improves when standing or sitting up
3. Labored or difficult breathing
7. Most carbon dioxide is transported to the lungs in this form.
8. The contribution of a single gas in a mixture of gases is called _____ pressure.
10. Reduced rate and depth of respirations

DOWN

2. Increased rate and depth of respirations
4. Temporary cessation of breathing
5. In the lungs, oxygen forms a weak bond with the iron portion of hemoglobin to form
   _____.
6. The process of carrying gases from the alveoli to the _____ and back is known as gas transport.
9. Hemoglobin releases oxygen in response to differences in _____ between arterial and venous blood.

List for Learning: Optimum Gas Exchange

List the three main factors necessary for optimum gas exchange.

1. _____

2. _____

3. _____

18
URINARY SYSTEM

Cells throughout the body continually perform a variety of metabolic processes, each of which results in waste products. The urinary system filters the blood to remove these products. But that's not all the kidneys do. They also regulate fluid volume, alter the levels of sodium and potassium, adjust the pH level, regulate blood pressure, and even contribute to the production of red blood cells. Complete the activities in this chapter to make sure you are well versed in all the functions of this body system.

Conceptualize in Color: **The Kidney**

Color the structures of the kidney in the following figure. Use the suggested colors or choose your own.

- Renal cortex: Brown
- Renal columns: Pink
- Renal pyramids: Green
- Renal papilla: Orange

- Minor calyces: Yellow
- Major calyces: Gold
- Renal pelvis: Red
- Ureter: Blue

Review your knowledge of the urinary system by completing the following crossword puzzle.

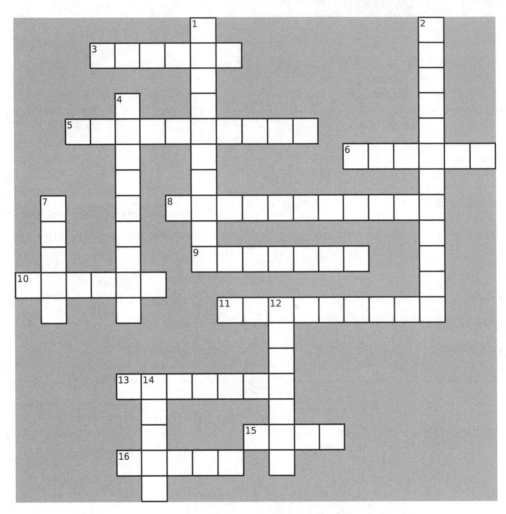

ACROSS

3. The renal _____ funnels urine from the calyces to the ureter.

5. Cluster of capillaries inside the renal corpuscle

6. Location in the kidney where renal corpuscles reside

8. Term for urination

9. Functional unit of the kidney

10. The part of the nephron where urine formation begins is the renal _____.

11. The process of eliminating waste from the body

13. Branch of medicine concerned with the urinary tract

15. Blood leaves the kidney through the renal _____.

16. This kidney sits lower than its mate

DOWN

1. Process by which substances pass from the glomerulus into Bowman's capsule

2. Common cause of kidney damage

4. The part of the nephron that filters blood plasma is the renal _____.

7. Blood vessels, the ureters, and nerves enter and leave the kidney through a slit called the _____.

12. Cup-like structures that collect urine leaving the renal papilla

14. Secreted by the kidney in response to low blood pressure

To more clearly understand the blood supply to nephrons, color the structures in the following figure. Use the suggested colors or choose your own.

- Afferent arteriole: Pink
- Efferent arteriole: Light red
- Glomerulus capillaries: Orange

- Peritubular capillaries: Dark red
- Veins that feed into renal vein: Blue

Next, draw arrows to show the direction of blood flow. Also, label the following structures:

- Proximal convoluted tubule
- Distal convoluted tubule

- Loop of Henle
- Collecting duct

Identify the structures of the nephron by coloring them as described here. Insert arrows to show the direction of flow.

- Afferent arteriole: Dark red
- Efferent arteriole: Blue
- Proximal convoluted tubule: Pink
- Descending limb of loop of Henle: Green
- Ascending limb of loop of Henle: Purple

- Distal convoluted tubule: Orange
- Collecting duct: Yellow
- Outline Bowman's capsule in brown
- Glomerulus: Light red

List for Learning: **Urine Formation**

List the three processes involved in urine formation.

1. _____

2. _____

3. _____

Glomerular Filtration

Review your knowledge of glomerular filtration by filling in the blanks in the following sentences. Choose from the words listed in the Word Bank. (Hint: Not all the words will be used.)

AFFERENT ARTERIOLE	**OSMOSIS**
BLOOD	**PLASMA PROTEINS**
EFFERENT ARTERIOLE	**PORES**
FILTRATION	**RENAL TUBULES**
GLOMERULAR FILTRATION RATE (GFR)	**WATER**
LOOP OF HENLE	**SMALL SOLUTES**

1. Blood flows into the glomerulus through the _____.

2. The walls of the glomerular capillaries are dotted with (a) _____,
allowing (b)_____ and (c)_____
to pass into Bowman's capsule through the process of (d)_____.
Cells that are too large to pass through include (e)_____ cells and
(f) _____.

3. Fluid in the Bowman's capsule flows into the (a) _____. The
amount of fluid filtered by the kidneys is called the (b)_____.

Renin-Angiotensin-Aldosterone System

A key mechanism for maintaining blood pressure and a steady glomerular filtration rate is the renin-angiotensin-aldosterone system. Describe the events, numbered 1 to 5 in the illustration, that occur in this system by writing in the numbered blanks. Then insert the name of the key hormone for each step in the boxes labeled A to D in the illustration.

1. A drop in blood pressure leads to decreased flow to the kidneys. This causes_____

_____

2. _____

_____

3. _____

_____

4. _____

_____

5. _____

_____

Tubular Reabsorption and Secretion

Clarify your understanding of tubular reabsorption and secretion by first coloring the structures of the renal tubule; use the colors suggested or choose your own. Then identify key substances reabsorbed or secreted along the various sections of the tubule. Write the symbol for each substance along the pertinent section with an arrow pointing out of the tubule to signify reabsorption and arrows pointing into the tubule to signify secretion. (Hint: Substances include H_2O, NaCl, K^+, H^+, glucose, urea, uric acid, NH_3, and drugs.) Insert arrows to depict the direction of flow within the tubule.

- Proximal convoluted tubule: Green
- Descending limb of the loop of Henle: Blue
- Ascending limb of the loop of Henle: Pink

- Distal convoluted tubule: Purple
- Collecting duct: Yellow

Unscramble the words on the left to discover the names of hormones acting on the renal tubule. Then draw lines to link the name of each hormone to its characteristics.

1. RELATEDSOON

— — — — — — — — — — —

2. LARIAT RACERINTUIT DIETPEP

— — — — — — — — — — — — — — —

— — — — — —

3. DRAINCUTIEIT EMHONOR

— — — — — — — — — — —

— — — — — —

4. HAIRDOPARTY HOMERNO

— — — — — — — — —

— — — — — — —

a. Inhibits the secretion of aldosterone and antidiuretic hormone

b. Causes the cells of the distal and collecting tubules to become more permeable to water; water flows into the interstitial fluid and urine volume decreases

c. Called the "salt-retaining hormone"

d. Secreted by the adrenal cortex in response to falling blood levels of Na^+ or rising blood levels of K^+

e. Secreted by the parathyroid glands in response to low blood calcium levels

f. Prompts the distal convoluted tubule to absorb more Na^+ and secrete more K^+

g. Secreted by atria of the heart in response to rising blood pressure

h. Causes blood volume to increase and blood pressure to rise

i. Secreted by the posterior pituitary gland (neurohypophysis)

j. Causes distal convoluted tubule to excrete more NaCl and water

k. Prompts the renal tubules to reabsorb more calcium and excrete more phosphate

In the following list, highlight the substances not normally found in urine. (The presence of these substances in urine indicates a disease process.)

Urea

Glucose

Blood

Uric acid

Ketones

Albumin

Ammonia

Hemoglobin

Creatinine

Urinary Bladder

Color the following structures in the figure below. Use the colors suggested or choose your own.

- Detrusor muscle: Pink
- Ureters: Brown
- Urethra: Green
- External urinary sphincter: Purple

- Internal urethral sphincter: Orange
- Trigone: Blue
- Rugae: Outline in black

Illuminate the Truth: **Renal Disorders**

Highlight the word or phrase that correctly completes each sentence.

1. Kidney stones often become lodged in the (urethra)(ureter).

2. Women are prone to bladder infections because of their relatively short (urethra)(ureter).

3. Diabetes insipidus results from (hyposecretion)(hypersecretion) of ADH, resulting in (excessive)(scant) urine output.

4. In acute renal failure, the kidneys (often resume normal function)(rarely resume normal function) following treatment.

5. (Chronic renal insufficiency)(Acute renal failure) often results from diseases such as diabetes or hypertension.

6. In chronic renal insufficiency, nephron damage is (extensive and irreversible)(limited and reversible).

19

FLUID, ELECTROLYTE, & ACID-BASE BALANCE

About two-thirds of the body consists of water. Dissolved within the water are thousands of substances, such as electrolytes, that are used in the body's biochemical reactions. The maintenance of homeostasis, and even life itself, depends upon a precise balance of water, electrolytes, and pH. Complete the activities in this chapter to gain a better understanding of this complex topic.

List for Learning: Fluid Compartments

Write the names of the four types of fluid that make up extracellular fluid.

1. _____
2. _____
3. _____
4. _____

List for Learning: Output

List the four ways fluid leaves the body.

1. _____
2. _____
3. _____
4. _____

Regulation of Intake and Output

Test your knowledge of the mechanisms used by the body to regulate intake and output by completing the following sentences.

Various factors, including excessive sweating, cause the volume of total body water to decline.

1. Blood pressure _____, sodium concentration _____,

and osmolarity _____.

2. Physical changes stimulate the thirst center in

the _____.

3. _____ decreases, causing a

dry mouth and a sensation of _____

_____.

4. Consumption of _____

leads to a _____ in total

water volume.

5. Physical changes stimulate the _____

_____, which stimulates

the posterior pituitary to secrete the hormone

_____.

6. The hormone _____ prompts the

kidneys to _____ more water and

produce _____ urine.

7. The rate of fluid loss _____.

Dehydration

Test your understanding of the fluid shifts that occur in dehydration by placing the following statements in the proper sequence. Do so by inserting a 1 by the sentence describing what would occur first, a 2 by the sentence describing what would occur next, and so on.

_____ **A.** Fluid shifts from tissues into the bloodstream.

_____ **B.** Water is lost through sweat.

_____ **C.** Fluid shifts from cells into tissues.

_____ **D.** Fluid moves from the bloodstream to the sweat glands.

_____ **E.** The osmolarity of the blood rises.

_____ **F.** The osmolarity of tissue fluid rises.

Unscramble the words on the left to discover the chief electrolytes in blood plasma. Draw a line to link each electrolyte to its characteristics.

1. MUDISO

— — — — — — —

2. AIMSTOUPS

— — — — — — — — —

3. LACCUMI

— — — — — — —

4. COLDHIRE

— — — — — — — —

5. HEATHSPOP

— — — — — — — — — —

a. The main electrolyte in extracellular fluid

b. Is retained or excreted along with sodium, so that an imbalance in this ion occurs along with a sodium imbalance

c. The terms *hyperkalemia* and *hypokalemia* refer to abnormal plasma concentrations of this ion.

d. Levels are primarily regulated by aldosterone and ADH

e. Besides strengthening bones, this ion plays a key role in muscle contraction, nerve transmission, and blood clotting.

f. The terms *hypernatremia* and *hyponatremia* refer to abnormal plasma concentrations of this ion.

g. Aldosterone (which is released in response to rising plasma levels of this ion) causes the kidneys to increase excretion of this ion.

h. The body can tolerate broad variations in the concentration of this ion.

i. The chief cation of extracellular fluid

j. The terms *hypercalcemia* and *hypocalcemia* refer to abnormal plasma concentrations of this ion.

k. An increased plasma concentration of this ion usually represents a water deficit.

l. High plasma levels of this ion can lead to fatal cardiac arrhythmias.

m. Influences how body water is distributed between fluid compartments

n. The most abundant extracellular anion

Regulation of Sodium

Complete the following sentences to clarify the mechanisms the body uses to regulate sodium and normalize serum osmolarity in situations involving water excess as well as water deficit. Choose from the words listed in the Word Bank. (Hint: Some words will be used more than once.)

ADH	FALL	SECRETE
ALDOSTERONE	INCREASE	SECRETION
CHLORIDE	INCREASED	SODIUM
CONSUMPTION	REABSORB	THIRST
DECREASE	RISE	WATER

WATER EXCESS

A water excess causes serum sodium levels to (1) _____. This causes serum osmolarity to (2) _____. The hormone (3) _____ then prompts renal tubules to reabsorb (4) _____. (5) _____ and (6) _____ are also reabsorbed.

The release of the hormone (7) _____ is suppressed, which causes the kidney to (8) _____ more water. Reabsorption of (9) _____, combined with the (10) _____ of water, causes serum sodium levels to (11) _____.

WATER DEFICIT

A water deficit causes serum sodium levels to (1) _____. This causes serum osmolarity to (2) _____. The hormone (3) _____ stimulates the kidneys to (4) _____ water.

At the same time, the hormone (5) _____ stimulates (6) _____ to promote water (7) _____. (8) _____ renal absorption of water combined with (9) _____ water intake causes serum sodium levels to (10) _____.

General Concepts of Fluids and Electrolytes

Highlight the correct word or phrase to complete each sentence.

1. The average daily fluid intake for an adult is (2500 mL)(1800 mL).

2. Water usually follows the movement of (potassium)(sodium).

3. pH reflects the concentration of (hydrogen ions)(bicarbonate ions) in the blood.

4. The body's normal pH range is (7.45 to 7.55)(7.35 to 7.45).

5. An acid (releases)(accepts) H^+ ions.

6. As the concentration of H^+ ions increases, the pH (increases)(decreases), and the solution becomes more (acidic)(alkaline).

7. (Physiological buffers)(Chemical buffers) are the first to respond to an acid-base imbalance.

8. When the body's pH drops, chemical buffers work by (binding)(releasing) H^+ ions.

9. A rising CO_2 level causes the concentration of H^+ ions to (decrease)(increase).

10. The (respiratory system)(renal system) is the slowest system to respond to an acid-base imbalance.

Respiratory Control of pH

The respiratory system helps the body maintain an appropriate pH. Review this process by completing the following sentences. Then follow the instructions to illustrate the process in the accompanying figures.

1. Central chemoreceptors in the _____ detect a fall in

   pH resulting from an accumulation of _____.
   (Insert symbols inside the small boxes in the accompanying figure to illustrate what is being described.)

2. The central chemoreceptors signal the _____

   centers to _____ the rate and depth of

   breathing. This results in the expulsion of _____.
   (Insert symbols in the small boxes in the accompanying figure to illustrate what is being described. Also, insert other arrows and symbols as appropriate to complete the illustration.)

3. Since less _____ is available to combine with water to

   form _____, the concentration of

   _____ falls and pH _____.
   (Insert symbols in the small boxes in the accompanying figure to illustrate what is being described.)

Fluid and Electrolytes

Test your knowledge of fluid and electrolyte principals by completing the following crossword puzzle.

ACROSS

2. When CO_2 levels are high, the kidneys reabsorb this to compensate.
7. Substances that break up into electrically charged particles when dissolved in water
11. Fluid deficiency that results when the body eliminates more water than sodium
12. Skin elasticity

DOWN

1. Cerebrospinal fluid and synovial fluid are categorized as _____ fluid.
3. Fluid between cells inside tissue
4. Volume depletion
5. Water produced as a byproduct of metabolic reactions is called _____ water.
6. This fluid makes up one component of extracellular fluid.
8. Persistence of pinched skin after release; a sign of dehydration
9. The kidneys are the only buffer system that expels this.
10. Occurs when fluid accumulates in interstitial spaces

Acid-Base Imbalances

One of the most important factors influencing homeostasis is the body's balance between acids and bases. An imbalance between acids and bases may result in acidosis or alkalosis. Test your ability to differentiate between these two conditions by highlighting the sentences pertaining to acidosis in pink and those pertaining to alkalosis in yellow.

1. May result from hypoventilation

2. May cause breathing to slow, so as to allow CO_2 to accumulate

3. May result from a loss of gastric juices, such as through vomiting or suctioning

4. Results from an excess concentration of H^+ ions in the plasma

5. Causes hypokalemia

6. Causes hyperkalemia

7. Produces symptoms of CNS depression, such as disorientation, confusion, and coma

8. Would result from a loss of CO_2

9. May trigger an increased rate of breathing so as to "blow off" CO_2

10. May result from diabetes mellitus

11. Caused by a loss of acid

12. Caused by a gain in acid

chapter 20
DIGESTIVE SYSTEM

Transforming food into fuel that the body can use is no simple task; it requires the use of a dozen organs, multiple enzymes, and thousands of chemical reactions. Use the activities in this chapter to help make sense of the digestive process.

Conceptualize in Color: Organs of the Digestive System

Color the organs of the digestive system in the figure below as follows:

- Esophagus: Pink
- Pharynx: Red
- Mouth: Tan
- Stomach: Yellow
- Liver: Brown
- Large intestine: Purple
- Small intestine: Orange
- Gallbladder: Green
- Salivary gland: Blue
- Pancreas: Outline in brown
- Rectum: Blue
- Anus: Pink

Color the layers of the digestive tract in the figure below as follows:

- Mucosa: Red
- Submucosa: Pink
- Muscularis: Orange
- Serosa: Yellow

Review the structures of the mouth, particularly as they relate to the digestive process, by filling in the blanks in the following sentences with the correct words or phrases. Then color each structure as described.

1. A key role of the tongue in digestion is to _____.
   (Color the tongue pink.)

2. A fold of mucous membrane called the _____ anchors the tongue
   to the floor of the mouth.
   (Color this structure red.)

3. The _____ separates the mouth from the nasal cavity.
   (Color this structure tan.)

4. The _____ forms an arch between the mouth and the

   nasopharynx.
   (Color this structure orange.)

5. The _____ hangs down from the soft palate.
   (Color this structure yellow.)

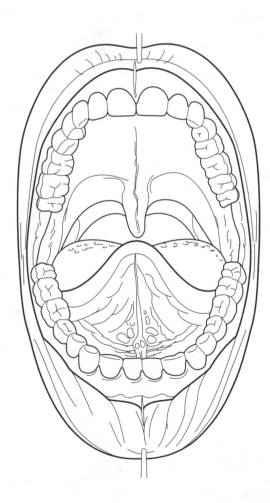

Fill in the blanks in the following sentences to link each of the main salivary glands with the region into which they drain. Then color each gland as described.

1. The _____ gland drains saliva to an area near the second upper molar.
   (Color this salivary gland purple.)

2. The _____ gland empties into the mouth on either side of the lingual frenulum.
   (Color this salivary gland orange.)

3. The _____ gland drains through multiple ducts onto the floor of the mouth.
   (Color this salivary gland green.)

Digestive System Basics

Fill in the following crossword puzzle to review some basic facts about the digestive system.

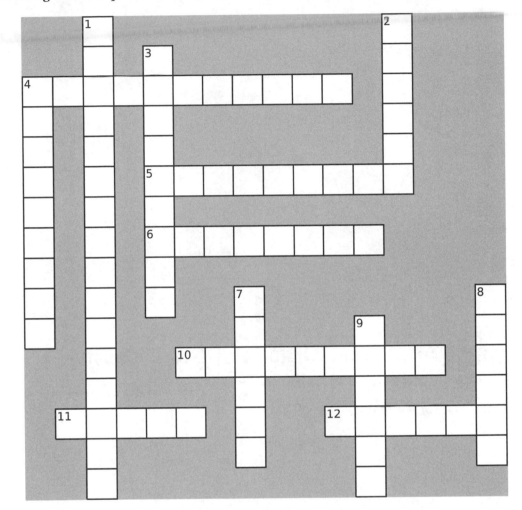

ACROSS

4. Chewing
5. Tissue layer of the digestive tract that contains glands, blood vessels, lymphatic vessels, and nerves
6. Chisel-like front teeth with sharp edges for cutting food
10. Early teeth that fall out and are replaced by permanent teeth
11. Mass of moistened food that can be swallowed easily
12. Pointed teeth designed to tear food

DOWN

1. The area of medicine concerned with the study of the digestive tract and the diagnosis and treatment of its diseases
2. Clear fluid secreted by the mouth that contains digestive enzymes
3. Process of breaking down food into a form that cells can use
4. Holds the intestines loosely in place
7. The mouth is also called the _____ cavity.
8. Hardest substance in the body
9. Teeth with flat surfaces for crushing or grinding food

List for Learning: **Organs of the Digestive Tract**

List the six organs of the digestive tract.

1. _____

2. _____

3. _____

4. _____

5. _____

6. _____

List for Learning: **Accessory Organs of the Digestive Tract**

List the six accessory organs of the digestive tract.

1. _____

2. _____

3. _____

4. _____

5. _____

6. _____

Color the structures of the tooth as described:

- Enamel. Light tan
- Dentin: Gold
- Pulp cavity: Red
- Cementum: Gray
- Periodontal ligament: Purple

- Gingiva: Pink
- Draw a red bracket around the crown
- Draw a green bracket around the root
- Draw an orange bracket around the neck
- Outline the root canal in black

Esophagus and Stomach

Fill in the blanks in the following sentences to describe the esophagus and stomach. Choose from the words listed in the Word Bank. (Hint: Not all the words will be used.)

CHIEF	PARIETAL	RUGAE	VITAMIN D
CHYME	PHARYNX	STOMACH	
LOWER ESOPHAGEAL SPHINCTER (LES)	POSTERIOR	TRACHEA	
OBLIQUE	PYLORIC	VITAMIN B12	

1. The esophagus extends from the _____ to the _____.

2. A muscular sphincter called the _____ prevents the backflow of stomach acid into the esophagus.

3. The esophagus lies _____ to the trachea.

4. The stomach contains folds in its lining called _____.

5. The muscularis of the stomach contains an additional layer of _____ muscle.

6. The stomach mixes particles of food with gastric juice to create a semifluid mixture called _____.

7. The _____ sphincter controls the opening between the stomach and duodenum.

8. _____ cells secrete hydrochloric acid as well as intrinsic factor, which is necessary for the absorption of _____.

9. _____ cells secrete digestive enzymes, such as pepsinogen.

The Stomach

In the figure below, color the regions of the stomach and nearby structures as follows:

- Cardia: Orange
- Fundus: Blue
- Body: Yellow
- Pylorus: Green
- Esophagus: Pink

- Duodenum: Tan
- Draw a red line along the lesser curvature
- Draw a purple line along the greater curvature
- Highlight pyloric sphincter in purple

Gastric Secretion

Fill in the blanks in the following sentences to describe the three phases of gastric secretion. Choose from the words listed in the Word Bank. (Hint: Words may be used more than once.)

CEPHALIC	**GASTRIN**	**INHIBIT**	**NEURAL**
GASTRIC	**INCREASE**	**INTESTINAL**	**PARASYMPATHETIC**

1. The sight, smell, taste, or thought of food sends (a) _____ impulses to the brain. The
   (b) _____ nervous system then signals the stomach to secrete (c) _____ juice
   as well as (d) _____. This is called the (e) _____ phase of gastric secretion.

2. When food enters the stomach, the (a) _____ phase begins. The stretching of the stomach
   triggers nervous impulses that (b) _____ the secretion of (c) _____
   juice and (d) _____.

3. As chyme moves into the duodenum, the (a) _____ phase begins. At this point, nervous
   impulses and hormones secreted by the duodenum (b) _____ gastric secretion.

The Liver

The figure below shows a posterior view of the liver. Color the structures of the liver as described.

- Right lobe: Light brown
- Left lobe: Dark brown
- Caudate lobe: Tan
- Quadrate lobe: Gold
- Falciform ligament: Gray

- Portal vein: Blue
- Hepatic artery: Red
- Inferior vena cava: Purple
- Gallbladder: Dark green
- Common hepatic duct: Light green

Posterior view

Fill in the blanks in the following sentences to describe the structure and function of hepatic lobules. Then color the figure as described.

1. Nutrient-rich blood from the stomach and intestine enters the lobule through small branches of the

   _____.
   (Color this structure dark blue.)

2. Oxygen-rich blood enters the lobule through small branches of the _____.
   (Color this structure red.)

3. The blood filters through the _____, allowing the cells to remove nutrients, hormones, toxins, and drugs.
   (Color these structures light blue. Insert arrow to show direction of flow.)

4. (a) _____ cells called (b) _____
   remove bacteria, worn-out red blood cells, and debris from the bloodstream.
   (Color these structures yellow.)

5. The _____ carries the processed blood out of the liver.
   (Color this structure purple.)

6. (a) _____ carry the bile secreted by hepatic cells and ultimately drain into the

   (b) _____.

Color the structures in the figure below as instructed.

- Right and left hepatic ducts: Blue
- Common hepatic duct: Purple
- Common bile duct: Light green
- Cystic duct: Yellow
- Gallbladder: Dark green
- Duodenum: Pink

- Pancreas: Gold
- Pancreatic duct: Orange
- Hepatopancreatic ampulla (ampulla of Vater): Mark with red dot
- Major duodenal papilla: Brown
- Hepatopancreatic sphincter (sphincter of Oddi): Black

Highlight the correct word or phrase to complete each sentence.

1. Most of the pancreas contains (endocrine)(exocrine) tissue.

2. (Acinar)(Duct) cells in the pancreas secrete digestive enzymes in an inactive form.

3. The enzymes are activated in the (stomach)(duodenum), after which they help break down lipids, proteins, and carbohydrates.

4. (Acinar)(Duct) cells in the pancreas secrete sodium bicarbonate, which buffers the acidic chyme entering the duodenum.

5. The arrival of chyme in the duodenum prompts the duodenum to secrete (cholecystokinin)(insulin), which (stimulates)(inhibits) the release of bile and pancreatic enzymes.

6. The hormone (gastrin)(secretin) also triggers gallbladder contraction and pancreatic enzyme secretion.

7. The hormone (gastrin)(secretin) causes the pancreatic ducts to release bicarbonate to neutralize the stomach acid.

The Small Intestine

In the figure below, color the regions of small intestine as instructed. Then use the same color to highlight the characteristics of each region. (For example, after coloring the duodenum green, highlight the sentences describing characteristics of the duodenum in green.)

- Duodenum: Green
- Ileum: Yellow
- Jejunum: Blue

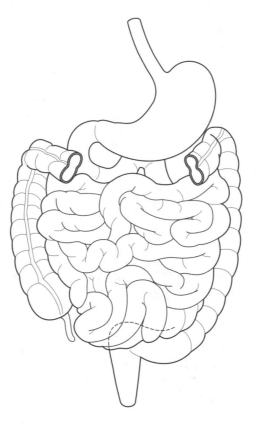

1. Begins at the pyloric valve and ends where the intestine turns abruptly downward

2. Forms the last 12 feet of intestine

3. Receives chyme from the stomach as well as pancreatic juice and bile

4. Is where stomach acid is neutralized and pancreatic enzymes begin the task of chemical digestion

5. Provides an ideal location for nutrient absorption

6. Forms the first 10 inches of small intestine

7. Wall of this part of the intestine is thick and muscular with a rich blood supply

8. Contains clusters of lymphatic nodules called Peyer's patches

9. Is where more digestive processes occur than in any other part of the intestine

Fill in the Gaps: Intestinal Wall

Fill in the blanks with the correct word or phrase to complete each sentence. Choose from the words in the Word Bank. (Hint: Not all of the words will be used. Also, some words may be used more than once.)

ACCELERATE	DECREASE	GOBLET	LACTEAL	SLOW
BILE	DIGESTIVE ENZYMES	HORMONES	MICROVILLI	VILLI
CHYME	EPITHELIAL	INCREASE	MUCUS	

1. The intestinal lining contains circular folds that _____ the progress of _____ and _____ its contact with the mucosa.

2. On top of the circular folds are projections called _____ .

3. These projections are covered by absorptive _____ cells as well as mucus-secreting _____ cells.

4. An arteriole, a venule, and a lymph vessel called a _____ fill the core of each villus.

5. The villi have a brush border of ultrafine _____ ; these projections serve to _____ the absorptive area and produce _____ .

Puzzle It Out: Digestive System Basics

Further your knowledge of key facts about the digestive system by completing the following crossword puzzle.

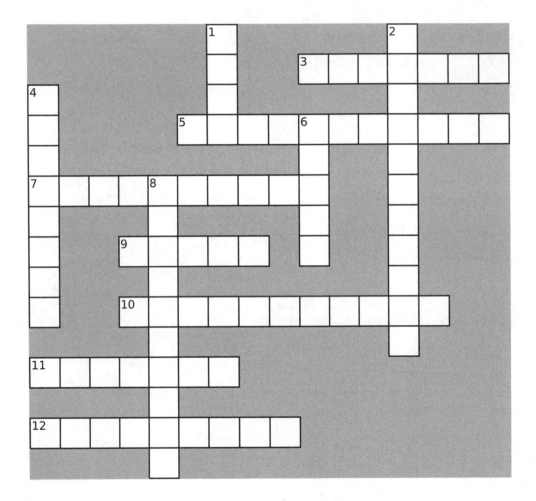

ACROSS

3. Term referring to the liver
5. Wave-like contractions that propel food through the digestive tract
7. Type of digestion that breaks food into smaller particles
9. Secretes bile
10. Sheets of hepatic cells that fan out from the center of the hepatic lobule
11. The portion of the mesentery that hangs over the small intestine like an apron is called the greater _____.
12. Main bile pigment

DOWN

1. Yellow-green fluid that aids in the digestion and absorption of fat
2. Serves to store and concentrate bile
4. Type of digestion that uses digestive enzymes to break down food particles into nutrients
6. The most important component of bile is bile _____.
8. Another name for the digestive tract is the _____ canal.

Carbohydrate Digestion

Describe the process of carbohydrate digestion by filling in the blanks in the following sentences with the correct word or phrase.

1. Salivary glands in the mouth secrete the enzyme _____, which works to hydrolyze _____ to _____.

2. The low pH of the stomach _____ the enzyme _____.

3. In the intestine, chyme mixes with _____ and the process of digestion _____.

4. The membranes of the cells covering the villi contain the enzymes _____, _____, and _____.

5. As chyme slides along the brush border, _____. This is called _____ digestion.

6. The final step in the digestion process produces _____, which is immediately absorbed.

Illuminate the Truth: **Protein Digestion**

Highlight the correct word or phrase to complete each sentence.

1. Enzymes called (proteases)(sucrases) work in the (mouth)(stomach) and (esophagus)(small intestine) to break peptide bonds.

2. In the stomach, the enzyme (pepsin)(amylase) hydrolyzes the peptide bonds between certain amino acids.

3. In the duodenum, the pancreatic enzymes (lipase and amylase)(trypsin and chymotrypsin) assume the task of breaking peptide bonds.

4. Brush border enzymes called (pepsin)(peptidases) break the remaining chains into individual amino acids, which are then absorbed into the bloodstream.

Test your knowledge of fat digestion by placing the following events in the proper sequence. Arrange the events by inserting numbers in the spaces provided. The first step has been provided to get you started.

___1___ **A.** A fat globule enters the duodenum.

_____ **B.** Pancreatic lipase begins to digest fat.

_____ **C.** Triglycerides travel through the lymphatic system and enter the bloodstream at the left subclavian vein.

_____ **D.** Glycerol and short-chain fatty acids are absorbed into the bloodstream of villi, and long-chain fatty acids are absorbed into the walls of the villi.

_____ **E.** Two substances in bile (lecithin and bile salts) emulsify fat.

_____ **F.** Fats are broken down into a mixture of glycerol, short-chain fatty acids, long-chain fatty acids, and monoglycerides.

_____ **G.** The gallbladder secretes bile.

_____ **H.** Triglycerides enter the lacteal of the villi.

Color the regions of the large intestine as instructed.

- Cecum: Pink
- Appendix: Green
- Ileocecal valve: Brown
- Ascending colon: Blue
- Transverse colon: Red
- Descending colon: Orange
- Sigmoid colon: Yellow
- Rectum: Tan
- Anal canal: Light blue
- Label the right colic (hepatic) flexure and the left colic (splenic) flexure

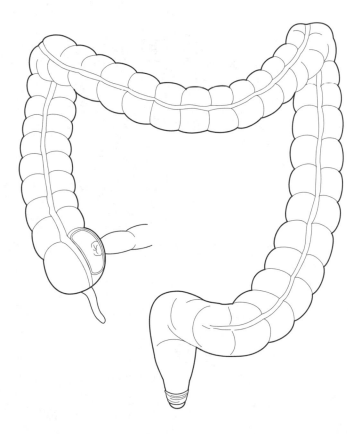

Large Intestine

Fill in the blanks with the correct word or phrase to complete each sentence. Choose from the words in the Word Bank. (Hint: Not all the words will be used.)

APPENDIX	**CHYME**	**FLATUS**	**NUTRIENTS**
BACTERIAL FLORA	**FECES**	**HAUSTRA**	**WATER**

1. The large intestine acts to absorb a large amount of _____ from food residue.

2. Pouches called _____ exist all along the large intestine.

3. The _____ contains masses of lymphoid tissue and serves as a source for immune cells.

4. The large intestine houses hundreds of bacteria called _____.

5. One of the products of bacterial action is intestinal gas, called _____.

6. Waste material that exits the large intestine is called _____.

21 NUTRITION & METABOLISM

The body's source of energy is food. However, before the body can access that energy, food must be broken down into usable components. In turn, those components must undergo chemical reactions within cells before that energy is unleashed. To ensure that you have a working knowledge of nutrition and metabolism, complete the activities in this chapter.

Make a Connection: **Carbohydrates**

Unscramble the words on the left to discover the names of the three forms of dietary carbohydrates. Then draw a line to link each form with its particular characteristics. (Hint: One characteristic is used more than once.)

1. AMECHANICSDOORS

   — — — — — — — — — — — — — — — — — —

2. CARDIACDISHES

   — — — — — — — — — — — — — — —

3. ACHILDCARESPOSY

   — — — — — — — — — — — — — — — —

a. Known as complex carbohydrates

b. Known as simple sugars

c. Broken down into monosaccharides during the digestive process

d. Consist of the starches found in vegetables, grains, potatoes, rice, and legumes

e. Taste sweet

f. Examples include fruit sugar as well as glucose and galactose

g. Examples include table sugar as well as the sugar found in milk

h. Are absorbed through the small intestine without being broken down

i. Includes cellulose

Nutrition Concepts

Improve your knowledge of some of the concepts of nutrition by completing the following crossword puzzle.

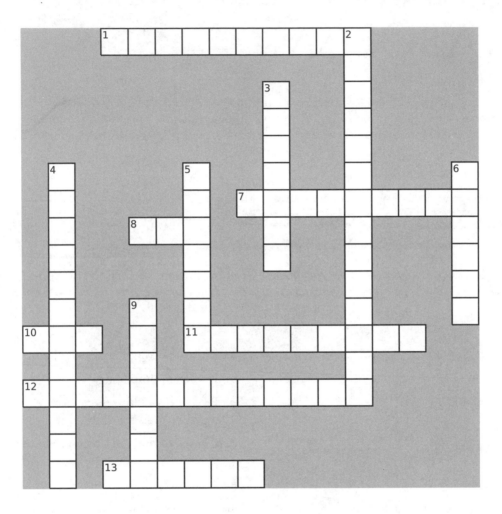

ACROSS

1. Chemical reactions occurring within cells that transform nutrients into energy
7. An important contributor of fiber in the diet
8. The amount of energy the body needs at rest (abbreviation)
10. Energy-dense nutrient containing 9 calories/gram
11. The digestive system breaks food into usable components called _____.
12. The body's primary energy source
13. One factor affecting basal metabolic rate

DOWN

2. Group of vitamins and minerals needed by the body in small quantities
3. Nutrient used in every aspect of cellular metabolism
4. Location of the control centers for hunger and satiety
5. Hormone that stimulates appetite
6. Hormone secreted by adipose tissue that suppresses appetite
9. The amount of heat needed to raise the temperature of 1 g of water by 1°C

Illuminate the Truth: Nutrition Basics

Highlight the words or phrase that correctly completes each sentence about some basic nutrition concepts.

1. (Protein)(Carbohydrates) should make up the greatest percentage of the diet.

2. Most of the carbohydrates consumed should be in the form of (simple sugars)(complex carbohydrates).

3. Excess carbohydrates are (stored in the body as fat)(converted into protein).

4. Carbohydrates, lipids, proteins, and water are called (macronutrients)(essential nutrients).

5. Saturated fats are derived mainly from (plants)(animals).

6. The most energy-dense nutrient is (protein)(fat).

7. (Unsaturated)(Saturated) fats tend to be solid at room temperature.

8. Hydrogenated oils, such as margarine, are (saturated)(unsaturated) fats.

9. All carbohydrates are eventually broken down into (glucose)(glycogen), which is then used as fuel for energy.

10. Fats that must be obtained through the diet—such as linoleic acid, which is a necessary part of the cell membrane—are called (essential fatty acids)(essential lipids).

Fill in the Gaps: Proteins

Proteins fulfill a vast array of functions in the body. Fill in the blanks with the correct word or phrase that completes each sentence about this vital nutrient. Choose from the words listed in the Word Bank. (Hint: Not all the words will be used.)

AMINO ACIDS	**COMPLETE PROTEINS**	**MOLECULES**
ANIMAL	**ESSENTIAL AMINO ACIDS**	**NONESSENTIAL AMINO ACIDS**
CAN	**INCOMPLETE PROTEINS**	**PLANT**
CANNOT		

1. During the process of digestion, proteins are broken down into their individual _____.

2. Foods that supply all the essential amino acids are called _____; these foods mainly come from _____ sources.

3. Foods that lack one or more essential amino acids are called _____; these foods mainly come from _____ sources.

4. The body _____ store extra amino acids.

5. Amino acids that can be synthesized by the body and, therefore, do not need to be consumed in the diet are called _____.

6. Amino acids that cannot be synthesized by the body and, therefore, must be consumed in the diet are called _____.

Illuminate the Truth: Vitamins and Minerals

The body requires a number of vitamins and minerals to function properly. Highlight the word or phrase that correctly completes each sentence about some of these essential nutrients.

1. (Vitamin C)(Vitamin A) aids in wound healing.

2. (Vitamin K)(Vitamin E) is necessary for normal blood clotting.

3. A deficiency of (vitamin A)(vitamin D) results in night blindness.

4. A deficiency of (folic acid)(vitamin D) results in rickets.

5. Pernicious anemia results from a deficiency of (vitamin B_{12})(vitamin B_6).

6. Besides being necessary for the formation of bones and teeth, calcium is also necessary for (carbohydrate digestion)(muscle contraction and relaxation).

7. (Iodine)(Iron) is necessary for hemoglobin production.

8. Folic acid is needed for (bone growth and development)(synthesis of DNA).

9. A potassium deficiency can lead to (softening of the bones)(abnormal cardiac rhythm).

List for Learning: Fat-Soluble Vitamins

Fat-soluble vitamins are absorbed with dietary fat, after which they are stored in the liver and fat tissues of the body. List the four fat-soluble vitamins.

1. _____

2. _____

3. _____

4. _____

Make a Connection: Metabolism

Nutrients are transformed through metabolism into energy the body can either use immediately or store for later use. Unscramble the words on the left to discover the two types of metabolic processes. Then draw lines to the list on the right to link each process to its particular characteristics.

1. ANIMALSOB

    _ _ _ _ _ _ _ _ _ _

2. BOATSCLAIM

    _ _ _ _ _ _ _ _ _ _

a. Used in protein metabolism

b. Breaks down complex substances into simpler ones or into energy

c. Forms complex substances out of simpler ones

d. Used in the metabolism of carbohydrates and lipids

Fill in the Gaps: Carbohydrate Metabolism

Test your knowledge of carbohydrate metabolism by filling in the blanks in the following sentences with the correct word or phrase. Choose from the words listed in the Word Bank. (Hint: Not all the words will be used.)

AEROBIC	**ANAEROBIC**	**GLYCOGEN**
AEROBIC RESPIRATION	**ANAEROBIC FERMENTATION**	**GLYCOLYSIS**
A FRACTION	**BURNED AS ENERGY**	**STORED**
ALL	**GLUCOSE**	

1. All ingested carbohydrates are converted to _____, most of which is immediately _____.

2. The first phase of carbohydrate metabolism is called _____; because it does not use oxygen, this is called an _____ process.

3. This first phase releases _____ of the available energy.

4. During a period of strenuous exercise, the next second phase of metabolism would be _____.

5. During a time of rest, the next phase of metabolism would be _____.

Anaerobic Fermentation

The process the body uses to metabolize carbohydrates varies according to the availability of oxygen. Test your knowledge of how the body metabolizes carbohydrates when oxygen is in short supply by filling in the blanks in the following sentences. Then illustrate the process by filling in the symbols to the left of each sentence with the name of the substances produced along the way

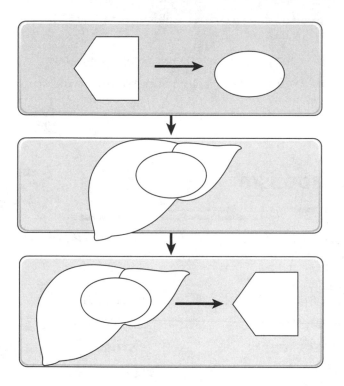

1. When oxygen is in short supply, _____ _____ is converted into _____.

2. The _____ then travels through the bloodstream to the _____ _____, where it is stored.

3. Later, during a period of rest when oxygen becomes available, _____ is converted into _____, which may then enter the series of reactions in _____.

Aerobic Respiration

Now test your knowledge of how the body metabolizes carbohydrates when oxygen is available by filling in the blanks in the following sentences. Then illustrate the process by filling in the symbols to the left of each sentence with the name of the substances produced along the way.

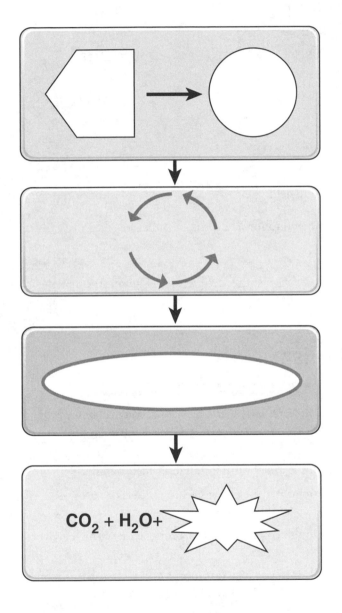

1. When oxygen is available, _____ _____ enters the _____ and is converted into _____.

2. This begins a series of reactions known as the _____.

3. This is followed by still another series of reactions called the _____ _____.

4. The end result is the complete breakdown of _____ into carbon dioxide, water, and, most importantly, large amounts of _____.

Lipid Metabolism

Review the process of lipid metabolism by filling in the blanks in the following sentences. Choose from the words listed in the Word Bank. (Hint: Not all the words will be used. Also, words may be used more than once.)

ACETYL CoA	**FATTY ACID(S)**	**LARGE**
ADIPOSE TISSUE	**GLUCOSE**	**SMALL**
CITRIC ACID	**GLYCOLYSIS**	**THE LIVER**
ELECTRON TRANSPORT		

1. When needed for energy, fat molecules stored within _____ are hydrolyzed into glycerol and three molecules of _____.

2. Glycerol enters the _____ pathway and yields a _____ amount of energy.

3. At the same time, _____ are broken down to form _____.

4. In turn, _____ proceeds through the _____ cycle and _____ chain to yield _____ amounts of energy.

Protein Metabolism

While carbohydrates and fat are mainly used to supply energy, proteins have a different role. Review some of the facts about protein metabolism by highlighting the word or phrase that correctly completes each sentence.

1. Proteins are mainly used to (supply energy)(build tissue); this is called protein (anabolism)(catabolism).

2. Protein (anabolism)(catabolism) is the process whereby proteins may be converted to glucose or fat or used directly as fuel.

3. During the digestion process, proteins are broken down into (glucose)(individual amino acids), which are then (stored as fat)(recombined to form new proteins).

4. Before proteins are used for energy, they are altered in the liver to produce (ammonia and keto acid)(urea and citric acid).

5. A nitrogenous waste product resulting from protein catabolism is (urea)(ketones).

Make a Connection: Thermoregulation

Unscramble the words on the left to discover three ways the body loses heat. Then draw lines to link each to its particular characteristics.

1. ARADIOTIN

— — — — — — — — —

2. TICCOONDUN

— — — — — — — — — —

3. AVIATORNOPE

— — — — — — — — — — —

a. Involves the transfer of heat between two materials that touch each other

b. Involves the transfer of heat through the air by electromagnetic heat waves

c. Uses heat to change water into a gas

d. How our bodies tend to lose heat

e. An example is standing in bright sunlight

f. An example is perspiration

g. An example is a warm chair after we stand from sitting

Illuminate the Truth: Regulation of Body Temperature

Several negative feedback mechanisms regulate body temperature. Refine your knowledge of these processes by highlighting the word or phrase that correctly completes each sentence.

1. The (pituitary gland)(hypothalamus) acts as the body's thermostat: it monitors the temperature of the (blood)(skin) and sends signals to blood vessels and sweat glands.

2. When the body temperature rises too high, the (hypothalamus)(pituitary gland) signals cutaneous blood vessels to (constrict)(dilate). More warm blood flows (close to the body's surface)(deep into the body) and heat is (lost)(conserved) through the skin.

3. If the temperature remains high, sweat glands produce sweat; in turn, the (production)(evaporation) of sweat produces (cooling)(warming).

4. When the body temperature falls below normal, the (pituitary gland)(hypothalamus) signals cutaneous blood vessels to (constrict)(dilate). More warm blood (flows to the body's surface)(remains confined deep in the body). As a result, (less)(more) heat is lost through the skin.

5. If the temperature remains below normal, the body begins to (shiver)(grow rigid). As a result, muscles (retain)(release) heat and the body's temperature (falls)(rises).

22
HUMAN
MICROBIOME

The human body houses a community of microbes that outnumber human cells 10 to 1. Discovery of this vast ecosystem is transforming how practitioners view both health and disease. Use the activities in this chapter to build upon your knowledge of the microbes that exist on, and in, the human body.

Illuminate the Truth: Facts about the Human Microbiome

Highlight the word or phrase that most accurately completes each sentence.

1. The human microbiome (is present at birth)(builds over time).

2. Scientists have learned that the inhabitants of specific bacterial communities—such as those in the mouth or intestines—(tend to be consistent)(often vary widely) between individuals.

3. (Bacteria)(Viruses) make up the bulk of the human microbiome.

4. The sinus passages of a person with sinusitis tend to contain (more)(fewer) species of bacteria as compared to the sinus passages of a person without sinusitis.

5. Children acquire significant components of their microbiomes (through their diet)(from their mothers).

Bacterial Structures

Identify the structures of bacteria by coloring the structures in the figure as suggested:

- Capsule: Green
- Cell wall: Orange
- Cytoplasmic membrane: Blue
- DNA: Pink

- Ribosomes: Red
- Plasmids: Brown
- Pilli: Purple
- Flagellum: Dark blue

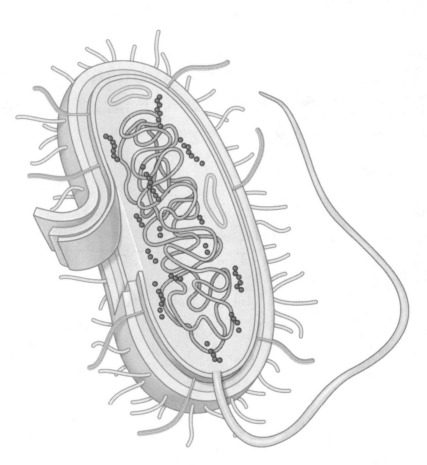

Improve upon your knowledge of bacterial structures by completing the sentences below. Choose the correct word or phrase from the Word Bank. (Hint: Some words may be used more than once; also, not all words or phrases will be used.)

CAPSULE	**PLASMIDS**
CELL WALL	**RESIST**
CYTOPLASMIC MEMBRANE	**RESPOND TO**
FLAGELLA	**THICK**
GROUPED IN THE CELL'S CENTRAL REGION	**THIN**
PILI	**WITHIN THE CELL'S NUCLEUS**

1. Some species of bacteria contain a gelatinous covering called a _____ that keeps the bacterium from drying out.

2. A rigid _____ encloses the bacterium and gives the cell its shape.

3. The _____ regulates the flow of materials into and out of the cell.

4. Because the composition of the _____ varies between species, it is an important distinguishing factor between bacterial types.

5. Many species of bacteria have small, hair-like projections called _____ that allow bacteria to attach to other cells and surfaces.

6. Small loops of bacterial DNA are called _____.

7. Some bacteria have _____, which aid in motility.

8. Bacterial DNA is found _____.

9. Bacterial structures that allow bacteria to trade genes are called _____.

10. Bacteria containing a _____ are more likely to cause disease.

11. Gram-positive bacteria have a _____ layer of peptidoglycan and tend to _____ antibiotic treatment.

Review the structures of viruses by coloring the structures in the figure below as suggested.

- Capsid: Blue
- Envelope: Orange
- Nucleic acid: Yellow
- Spikes: Brown

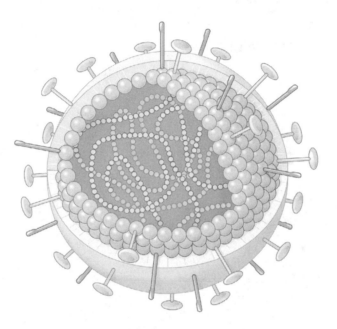

Unscramble the following words to discover the three basic viral shapes. Then draw a line to link each shape to its particular characteristics.

1. LCIHAEL

  — — — — — — —

2. YHLLRDOPAE

  — — — — — — — — —

3. CPLMXOE

  — — — — — — —

a. Adenovirus has this shape

b. Rabies virus has this shape

c. Is a protein cylinder

d. A bacteriophage has this shape

e. Consists of many triangular faces

Viral Replication

Viral replication occurs rapidly: a single cell may produce from 10,000 to 50,000 new viruses in as little as 48 hours. Test your knowledge of how this occurs by describing the process in the spaces below. Use the figure provided for clues. To further solidify your knowledge, color the figures using colors of your own choosing.

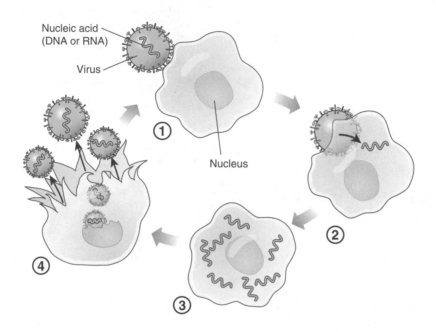

Nucleic acid (DNA or RNA)

Virus

Nucleus

1. _____

2. _____

3. _____

4. _____

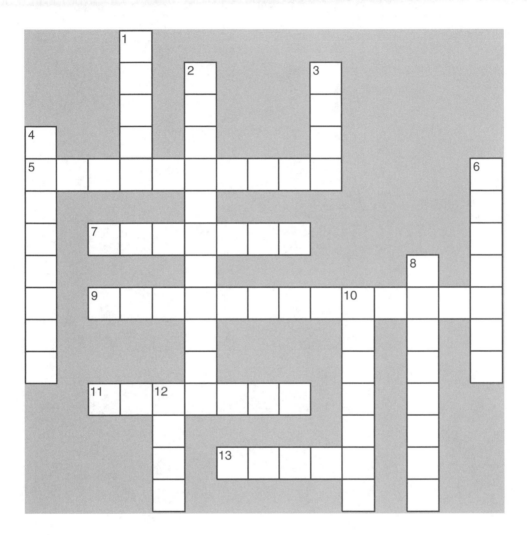

Puzzle it Out: Microbiome Facts

Complete the following crossword puzzle to review key facts about the human microbiome.

ACROSS

5. Interferes with a bacterium's ability to manufacture peptidoglycan
7. Bacteria having a rod shape
9. Complex virus that attaches to the surface of a cell before injecting its nucleic acid into the target cell
11. Structure that allows bacteria to ward off white blood cells
13. Molds and yeasts

DOWN

1. Round bacteria
2. Frequent culprit in microbiome disruption
3. Place on the body where fungal infections often begin
4. Spiral-shaped bacteria
6. Bacteria lack this
8. Microorganism known to cause disease
10. Bacterial structure that allows bacteria to be extremely adaptable
12. Gram-negative bacteria stain this color

23
REPRODUCTIVE SYSTEMS

In human reproduction, sex cells from the male and the female fuse to create a genetically unique individual. Structurally, the male and female reproductive systems differ significantly. Build upon your knowledge of these two systems by completing the activities in this chapter.

Make a Connection: Accessory Glands

The male reproductive system includes three sets of accessory glands. Unscramble the words on the left to discover the names of these glands. Then draw lines to link each gland to its particular characteristics.

1. LANESIM SECVILE

   _ _ _ _ _ _ _ _ _ _ _ _ _ _ _ _

2. SPARETOT DALNG

   _ _ _ _ _ _ _ _ _ _ _ _ _

3. HARBOURBULLET LAGND

   _ _ _ _ _ _ _ _ _ _ _ _ _ _ _ _

   _ _ _ _ _

a. Secretes a clear fluid into the penile portion of the urethra during sexual arousal

b. Encircles urethra and ejaculatory duct

c. Secretes a thick, yellowish fluid into the ejaculatory duct

d. Fluid secreted comprises about 30% of the fluid portion of semen

e. Fluid secreted comprises about 60% of semen

f. Fluid secreted serves as a lubricant during intercourse and also neutralizes the acidity of residual urine in the urethra

g. Secreted fluid contains fructose as well as other substances that nourish sperm and help ensure motility

h. Secretes a thin, milky, alkaline fluid into the urethra

Reproductive Terms

Test your knowledge of some terms specific to the reproductive system by completing the following crossword puzzle.

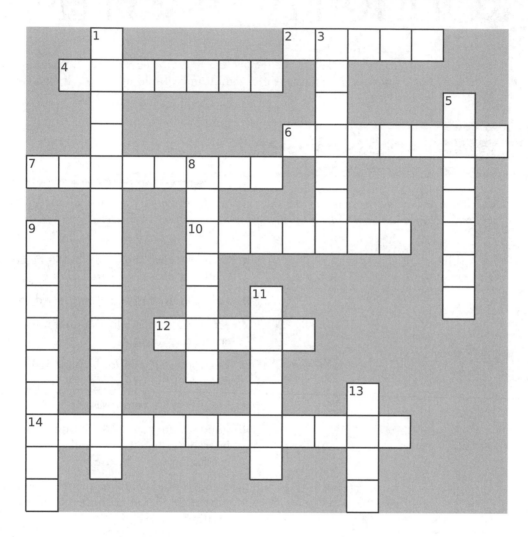

ACROSS

2. Term for the primary sex organ
4. Male structure that serves both the reproductive and urinary systems
6. Foreskin
7. Hormone necessary for the development of female secondary sex characteristics
10. Process by which gametes divide
12. Whitish fluid emitted during ejaculation that contains both sperm and the secretions of the accessory glands
14. Male hormone necessary for sperm production and the development of male secondary sex characteristics

DOWN

1. Undescended testes
3. Primary sex organs in females
5. Sac of tissue in which the testes lie
8. Sex cells
9. Muscle that contracts in cold weather to pull the testes closer to the body
11. Primary sex organs in males
13. Secretion of this hormone by hypothalamus marks the onset of puberty

Fill in the blanks in the following sentences to correctly describe the structure and function of the testes. Then color the figure as suggested to enhance your learning.

1. A strand of connective tissue called the _____ extends from the abdomen to each testicle; housed inside are blood, lymphatic vessels, and nerves. *(Color this structure gray.)*

2. Fibrous tissue separates each testis into more than 200 _____. *(Outline these areas in brown.)*

3. Coiled inside each of these structures are one to three tightly coiled ducts called _____, which is where sperm are _____. *(Color these structures yellow.)*

4. A network of vessels called the _____ lead away from this area and provide a location in which sperm partially mature. *(Color these vessels blue.)*

5. _____ ductules conduct immature sperm away from the testes. *(Color these vessels green.)*

6. Sperm pass into the _____, where they remain fertile for 40 to 60 days. *(Color this structure orange.)*

7. Sperm leave the previous structure and pass into the _____. *(Color this structure purple.)*

Color the structures of the male reproductive system in the following figure. Use the colors suggested or choose your own.

- Vas deferens: Dark blue
- Ejaculatory duct: Fuschia
- Bulbourethral gland: Brown
- Seminal vesicle: Yellow
- Prostate gland: Light green
- Urethra: Purple
- Testis: Gray
- Epididymis: Gold

- Scrotum: Tan
- Corpus spongiosum: Red
- Corpus cavernosum: Pink
- Glans penis: Orange
- Prepuce: Dark green
- Urinary bladder: Light blue

Thousands of sperm are produced each second. Insert numbers in the spaces provided to arrange the events of spermatogenesis in the proper order.

_____ **A.** Daughter cells of spermatogonia differentiate into slightly larger cells called primary spermatocytes, which move toward the lumen of the seminiferous tubule.

_____ **B.** Spermatids differentiate to form heads and tails and eventually transform into mature spermatozoa (sperm), each with 23 chromosomes.

_____ **C.** Each secondary spermatocyte divides to form two spermatids.

_____ **D.** Spermatogonia in the walls of the seminiferous tubules divide by mitosis to produce two daughter cells, each with 46 chromosomes.

_____ **E.** Through meiosis, the primary spermatocyte yields two genetically unique secondary spermatocytes, each with 23 chromosomes.

More Reproductive Facts

Highlight the word or phrase that correctly completes each sentence.

1. The most common cancer in American men is (prostate)(testicular) cancer.

2. The body of the penis is called the (shaft)(prepuce).

3. Through the process of meiosis, each daughter cell has (46)(23) chromosomes.

4. Each daughter cell of meiosis is (genetically identical to)(genetically unique from) the parent cell.

5. An important quality of semen is its (acidity)(alkalinity).

6. The portion of sperm that contains genetic information is the (acrosome)(head).

7. The portion of the sperm that contains an enzyme that helps it penetrate an egg is the (acrosome)(middle piece).

8. The testes are located outside the body to (protect them from infection)(keep them cooler).

List for Learning: **Sexual Response**

Using the spaces provided, list the four phases of both the male and female sexual response.

1. _____

2. _____

3. _____

4. _____

Female Reproductive System

Color the structures of the female reproductive system in the following figure. Use the colors suggested or choose your own.

- Uterus: Red
- Fallopian tube: Pink
- Ovary: Gray
- Cervix: Orange
- Rectum: Brown

- Vagina: Purple
- Bladder: Blue
- Labium majus: Tan
- Labium minus: Gold
- Urethra: Light blue

Unlike the male, the organs of the female reproductive system are housed within the abdominal cavity. Review these structures by filling in the blanks in the following sentences. Then follow the instructions to color the structures in the figure below.

1. The narrow portion of the fallopian tube closest to the uterus is called the _____; the middle portion is called the _____, while the funnel-shaped distal portion is called the

   _____.
   (Color the fallopian tubes pink.)

2. Finger-like projections called _____ fan over the ovary.
   (Color these structures orange.)

3. The uterus is held in place by the _____ ligament.
   (Color this structure tan.)

4. The curved, upper portion of the uterus is called the _____.
   (Outline this portion in blue.)

5. The inferior end of the uterus is called the _____.
   (Color this structure brown.)

6. The _____ serves as a receptacle for the penis and sperm and as a route for the discharge of menstrual blood.
   (Color this structure purple.)

7. The smooth muscle layer of the uterus is called the _____.
   (Color this structure light red.)

8. The innermost layer of the uterus, called the _____, is where an embryo attaches.
   (Color this structure dark red.)

Color the structures of the breasts. Use the colors suggested or choose your own.

- Pectoralis muscle: Pink
- Acini: Red
- Lobules: Outline in purple
- Lactiferous ducts: Tan

- Lactiferous sinuses: Orange
- Areola: Brown
- Adipose tissue: Yellow
- Suspensory ligaments: Blue

Puzzle It Out: Female Reproductive System

Enhance your knowledge of some of the terms specific to the female reproductive system by completing the following crossword puzzle.

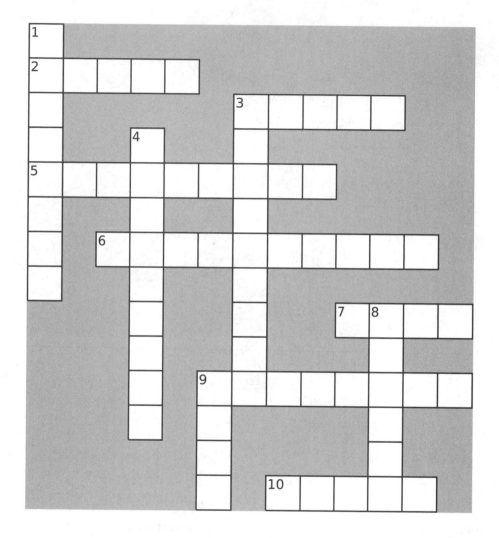

ACROSS

2. Thick folds of skin and adipose tissue on either side of the vaginal opening are called the _____ majora.
3. Collective term for female external genitalia
5. Process through which a mature ovum is formed
6. Cells surrounding the egg
7. The central region of the uterus
9. First menstrual period
10. Fold of mucous membrane partially covering the entrance to the vagina

DOWN

1. Small mound of erectile tissue in females that resembles a penis
3. Area inside the labia
4. State of life when menstruation ceases permanently
8. Another name for egg
9. Mound of hair-covered adipose tissue overlying the symphysis pubis is called the _____ pubis.

*A woman's reproductive system undergoes cyclical changes each month as it prepares for the possibility of pregnancy. These changes, called the reproductive cycle, consist of two interrelated cycles: the ovarian cycle and the menstrual cycle. Test your knowledge of the sequence of events of the ovarian cycle by filling in the blanks in the following sentences. Choose from the words listed in the Word Bank. (**Hint:** Words may be used more than once.)*

ANTERIOR	**FOLLICULAR**	**PROGESTERONE**
CORPUS ALBICANS	**FSH**	**LH**
CORPUS LUTEUM	**GONADOTROPIN-RELEASING HORMONE (GnRH)**	**LUTEAL**
ESTROGEN	**POSTERIOR**	

1. Low levels of _____ and _____ stimulate the hypothalamus to

    release _____ .

2. The hormone _____ stimulates the _____ pituitary to release the hormones

    _____ and _____ .

3. The hormone _____ triggers several follicles in the ovary to resume development, beginning

    what is known as the _____ phase.

4. As the follicle develops, it secretes _____ , which stimulates the thickening of the endometrium,

    as well as small amounts of _____ .

5. At the mid-point of the cycle, _____ levels peak, triggering a spike in _____ ,
    which causes ovulation.

6. The remnants of the follicle remain on the ovary and form the _____ , which marks

    the beginning of the _____ phase.

7. The _____ secretes large amounts of the hormone _____ and

    small amounts of _____ .

8. If fertilization doesn't occur, the _____ degenerates into inactive scar tissue called

    the _____ .

9. Levels of _____ and _____ plummet, causing the endometrium to
    slough off, resulting in menstruation.

Unscramble the words on the left to discover the names of the four phases of the menstrual cycle. Then draw a line to link each phase to its particular characteristics.

1. LAMETURNS

— — — — — — — — —

2. FIRETRAPOLIVE

— — — — — — — — — — — — —

3. CRYTOERES

— — — — — — — —

4. MANTLEPURSER

— — — — — — — — — — — —

a. Involves the atrophy of the corpus luteum

b. Blood vessels grow as the base layer is repaired

c. Time when menstruation occurs

d. Involves ischemia and necrosis of the endometrium

e. Dominated by increased levels of progesterone

f. Involves the shedding of the endometrium's functional layer

g. Encompasses days 26 to 28 of the cycle

h. Encompasses days 6 to 14 of the cycle

i. Rising levels of estrogen dominate

j. Encompasses days 15 to 26 of the cycle

k. Encompasses days 1 to 5 of the cycle

l. Involves increased thickening of the endometrium as it becomes suitable for implantation of a fertilized egg

m. Instituted by plummeting levels of progesterone

24
PREGNANCY & HUMAN DEVELOPMENT

The creation of a new life—beginning with the fusion of an egg and a sperm and culminating with the entrance of a neonate into the world—involves numerous body processes. Review some of these processes by completing the activities in this chapter.

Drawing Conclusions: Fertilization

Conception occurs when an egg and a sperm fuse. Strengthen your understanding of the fertilization process by filling in the blanks to complete the sentences. Then follow the instructions to color and label the figure on the next page.

1. As hundreds of sperm swarm the egg, the _____ on their heads release _____ that break down the cells and a gel-like layer called the _____ surrounding the egg.
   (Color the body of the sperm gray; the heads of the sperm yellow; the covering over the heads of the sperm green; the ganulosa cells tan; the gel-like coating of the egg blue; and the substance released from the heads of the sperm pink.)

2. A path is created that allows _____ (*Hint*: a number) sperm to penetrate the egg.
   (Label the sperm being blocked, the two sperm that are helping to clear a path into the egg, and the sperm that has penetrated the egg.)

3. As fertilization occurs, the _____ of the sperm is released into the ovum as its _____ degenerates and falls away.
   (Label the sperm that is fertilizing the egg.)

4. The _____ of the sperm, which has _____ chromosomes, fuses with the _____ of the egg, which also has _____ chromosomes, creating a single cell with _____ chromosomes.

5. The fertilized egg is called a _____.

Drawing Conclusions: Fertilization to Implantation

Fill in the blanks in the sentences to describe what occurs between fertilization and implantation. Then follow the instructions to draw the product of conception in each stage of development as it proceeds through the fallopian tube.

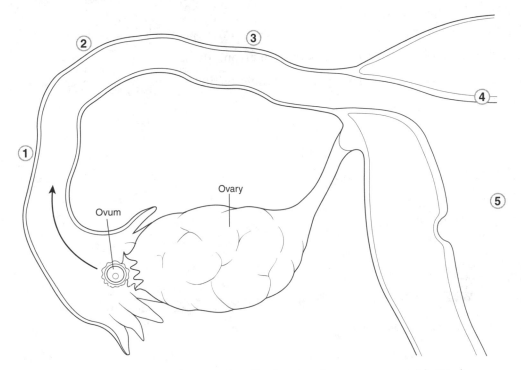

1. The _____ stage begins when fertilization forms a zygote with 23 chromosomes.
   (By the number 1 in the illustration, draw the egg being fertilized.)

2. Within 24 to 36 hours, the zygote divides by the process of _____ to form two daughter

   cells called _____.
   (By the number 2 in the illustration, draw this process using two separate figures. Label these figures.)

3. The divisions continue, with the cells _____ with each division. Finally, a blackberry-like

   cluster of (*Hint*: a number) _____ cells called a _____ results.
   (Draw this process by the number 3 in the illustration, using three separate figures. Label the final figure.)

4. Three to four days after fertilization, the morula enters the uterine cavity, where it _____

   for 2 or 3 days. As the cell cluster continues to divide, a hollow cavity forms; the cell cluster is now called a

   _____. This differentiates into two layers: an outer layer of cells called the

   _____, which eventually forms the _____, and an inner cell

   mass that becomes the _____.
   (Draw and label this structure by the number 4 in the illustration.)

5. About 6 days after ovulation, the _____ lands on and attaches to the endometrium—a

   process called _____.
   (Draw what is being described, using the space by the number 5 in the illustration.)

As the blastocyst attaches to the endometrium, it undergoes rapid changes. Highlight the word or phrase in each sentence to correctly describe these changes.

1. Shortly after implantation, the outer wall of the blastocyst, called the (trophoblast)(blastomere), fuses with the underlying endometrium.

2. About that time, the inner cell mass separates to create a narrow space called the (yolk sac)(amniotic cavity).

3. The inner cell mass flattens to form the (ectoderm)(embryonic disc).

4. Next, the (embryonic disc)(trophoblast) gives rise to three (germ layers)(embryonic layers), which produce the body's organs and tissues.

List for Learning: Germ Layers

Using the spaces provided, write the names of the three germ layers.

1. _____

2. _____

3. _____

Human Growth and Development Terms

Complete the crossword puzzle to test your understanding of terms used in human growth and development.

ACROSS

4. Stage of development beginning at fertilization and lasting for 16 days

5. The 3-month periods dividing the term of pregnancy

9. Transparent sac filled with fluid that surrounds the embryo and fetus

13. Extraembryonic membrane that serves as the foundation for the umbilical cord

14. Supplies the fetus with oxygen and nutrients during pregnancy

15. Fertilized egg

DOWN

1. Outermost membrane that surrounds other extraembryonic membranes

2. The union of the nuclei of the egg and sperm

3. Hormone that prompts the corpus luteum to secrete estrogen and progesterone and also forms the basis for pregnancy tests (*Hint*: use initials)

6. Stage of development lasting from the third until the eighth week of pregnancy

7. Fine hair covering the fetus' body

8. The time of growth before birth is called the _____ period.

10. Length of time from conception until birth

11. Process by which the fertilized cell divides by mitosis

12. Stage of development beginning the eighth week and lasting until birth

Stages of Prenatal Development

The approximately 9-month period between fertilization and birth transforms a single cell into a complete human being. Test your knowledge of the events that occur in each stage by highlighting the events of the pre-embryonic stage in pink, the events of the embryonic stage in blue, and the events of the fetal stage in yellow.

1. Formation of the amnion, yolk sac, allantois, and chorion

2. Begins at fertilization

3. Involves rapid growth

4. Differentiation of germ layers into organs and organ systems

5. Fusion of the trophoblast with the endometrium

6. Movement that can be felt by the mother occurs

7. Formation of the amniotic cavity

8. Begins sixteen days after conception and lasts for 6 weeks

9. Formation of the embryonic disc

10. Begins the eighth week and lasts until birth

11. Development of the placenta and umbilical cord

12. Formation of the three germ layers

13. Encompasses the time of the zygote

14. The heart begins to beat

Embryonic and Fetal Membranes

Learn to differentiate between the various membranes surrounding the embryo and fetus by coloring them as described.

- Uterus: Pink
- Chorion: Green
- Amnion: Orange

- Amniotic fluid: Blue
- Umbilical cord: Gray

- Yolk sac: Yellow
- Chorionic villi: Red

Because the fetus depends on the placenta for oxygen and nutrients as well as for the removal of waste products, the circulatory system of the fetus differs significantly from that of a newborn infant. Trace the pathway of fetal circulation by coloring the structures in the following figure as described.

1. Color the umbilical vein red to depict the oxygen-rich blood flowing in from the placenta.

2. Color the ductus venosus red as it bypasses the liver; change the color to purple as blood merges into the inferior vena cava. Draw a black arrow depicting the movement of blood from the umbilical vein, through the ductus venosus, and into the inferior vena cava.

3. Color blood in the right atrium purple; continue coloring into the left atrium and through the foramen ovale. Insert a black arrow depicting the movement of blood through foramen ovale.

4. Color the right ventricle purple; extend the purple color into the pulmonary trunk. Insert black arrows showing the movement of blood into the right ventricle and into the pulmonary trunk. Then show the passage of blood into the ductus arteriosus and the descending aorta by coloring these areas purple and inserting arrows.

5. Continue the purple color into the iliac and umbilical arteries. Insert black arrows to depict the flow of blood into the umbilical arteries and back to the placenta.

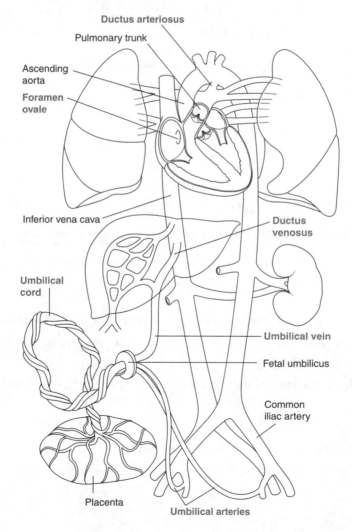

Childbirth

*Test your knowledge of the events occurring during childbirth by filling in the blanks to complete each sentence correctly. Choose from the words listed in Word Bank. (**Hint:** Not all the words will be used. Also, some words may be used more than once.)*

AFTERBIRTH	**EFFACEMENT**	**OXYTOCIN**	**SECOND**
BRAXTON-HICKS	**ESTROGEN**	**PROGESTERONE**	**THIRD**
DILATION	**FIRST**	**PSEUDO-CONTRACTIONS**	

1. The onset of labor is thought to result from a decline in the hormone _____ and an increase in the hormones _____ and _____.

2. The contractions sometimes known as "false labor" are called _____ contractions.

3. The _____ stage of labor is the longest.

4. The first stage of labor involves thinning of the cervical walls, called cervical _____, as well as progressive widening of the cervix, called cervical _____.

5. The baby is born during the _____ stage of labor.

6. The amniotic sac usually breaks during the _____ stage of labor.

7. The final stage of labor involves delivery of the _____.

Mammary Glands

After childbirth, the mammary glands produce and secrete milk to nourish the neonate. Review this process by highlighting the correct word or phrase in each of the following sentences.

1. The process by which the mammary glands produce and secrete milk is called (parturition)(lactation).

2. The growth of ducts throughout the mammary glands is stimulated by the high levels of (progesterone)(estrogen) during pregnancy.

3. The development of acini at the ends of the ducts is stimulated by the high levels of (estrogen)(progesterone) during pregnancy.

4. The production of milk is initiated by the secretion of (prolactin)(progesterone).

5. The secretion of the hormone (estrogen)(oxytocin) causes milk to be released into the ducts.

6. Before milk is secreted, the mammary glands secrete a yellowish fluid called (vernix caseosa)(colostrum).

25
HEREDITY

The process of passing traits from biological parents to children is called heredity, while the study of heredity is called genetics. Test your knowledge of this fascinating topic by completing the activities in this chapter.

Illuminate the Truth: Basic Heredity

Review some basic heredity concepts by highlighting the correct word or phrase in each of the following sentences.

1. Gametes contain (23)(46) chromosomes.

2. Chromosomes consist of long strands of tightly coiled (DNA)(genes).

3. Both males and females need (one normal Y chromosome)(one normal X chromosome).

4. X-linked recessive traits typically express themselves in (females)(males).

5. Trisomy 21 results from (nondisjunction)(mutation) of a chromosome.

6. The 23rd pair of chromosomes are (autosomes)(sex chromosomes).

7. Many common diseases result from an interaction between genetic mutations and (hormonal)(environmental) influences.

8. When homologous chromosomes have different alleles at a particular site, the person is said to be (homozygous)(heterozygous) for that trait.

Heredity Terms

Complete the following crossword puzzle to review some of the key terms associated with the study of genetics and heredity.

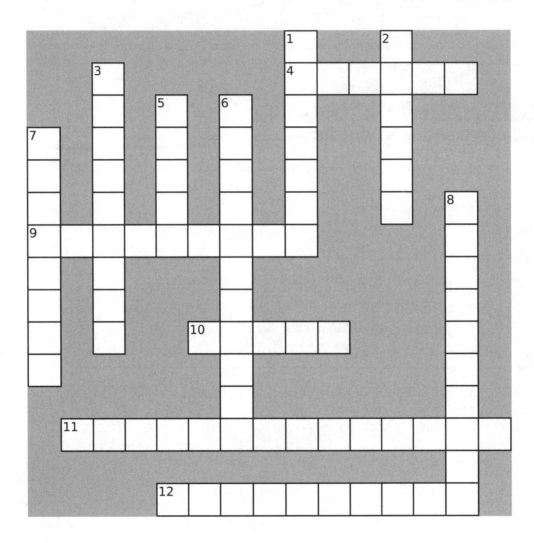

ACROSS

4. An alternative form of a gene
9. Non-sex chromosomes
10. The location of a gene on a specific chromosome
11. When homologous chromosomes fail to separate during meiosis
12. When an individual has two alleles that are the same, he is said to be _____ for the trait.

DOWN

1. These are the only cells that contain a single set of 23 chromosomes.
2. A complete set of genetic information for one person
3. Chart showing all the chromosomes arranged in order by size and structure
5. Contain the traits that each person inherits
6. DNA is spiraled into packages called _____.
7. A permanent change in genetic material
8. Name for similar-looking matched chromosomes

Insert the symbols for X and Y chromosomes by each of the male and female figures to symbolize their gender. Then draw arrows from each parent to each offspring to show how those chromosomes are transmitted. (One arrow and chromosome is inserted to get you started.)

Female child

Male child

Dominant and Recessive Genes

*Review the transmission of dominant and recessive traits by filling in the blanks in the following sentences. Choose from the words listed in the Word Bank. (**Hint:** Words may be used more than once.)*

BLUE	CODOMINANT	HOMOZYGOUS	WILL
BOTH	DOMINANT	NEITHER	WILL NOT
BROWN	HETEROZYGOUS	RECESSIVE	

1. A _____ allele overshadows the effect of a _____ allele.

2. If only one chromosome carries a dominant allele, the offspring _____ express the trait.

3. If only one chromosome carries a recessive allele, the offspring _____ express the trait.

4. When an allele for brown eyes is paired with an allele for blue eyes, the offspring (who is _____ _____ for the trait) will have _____ eyes.

5. When an allele with brown eyes is paired with another allele for brown eyes, the offspring (who is _____ _____ for that trait) will have _____ eyes.

6. When an allele with blue eyes is paired with another allele for blue eyes, the offspring (who is _____ _____ for that trait) will have _____ eyes.

7. Alleles that are equally dominant are called _____; in this instance, _____ alleles are expressed.

Sex-linked Inheritance

Highlight the correct word or phrase to complete each sentence.

1. Almost all sex-linked traits are (dominant)(recessive).

2. Sex-linked traits are carried on the (X)(Y) chromosome.

3. A common sex-linked disorder is (Down syndrome)(red-green color blindness).

4. If a female inherits the allele for a sex-linked disorder, she will (develop the disorder)(be a carrier of the disorder).

5. If a male inherits the allele for a sex-linked disorder, he will (develop the disorder)(be a carrier of the disorder).

Conceptualize in Color: # Autosomal Dominant Inheritance

Review the process of autosomal dominant inheritance by coloring the following figures. In this instance, the father is affected and the mother is unaffected. To illustrate the transmission of the disorder from the father to his children, color the figures as described.

- Dominant, affected gene: Red
- Recessive gene: Blue
- Everyone affected by the disorder: Red

- Unaffected people: Blue
- Carriers of the disorder: Purple

Review the process of autosomal recessive inheritance by coloring the following figures. In this instance, both parents are carriers of a trait. To illustrate the transmission of the disorder from the parents to their children, color the figures as described.

- Dominant, affected gene: Red

- Recessive gene: Blue

- Everyone affected by the disorder: Red

- Unaffected people: Blue

- Carriers of the disorder: Purple

*(**Hint:** Since both parents are carriers, each will have one red and one blue gene.)*

*Nondisjunction, which can affect sex chromosomes as well as autosomal chromosomes, is a common cause of genetic disorders. Use the space provided to illustrate the process of nondisjunction, with the end result being that one cell exhibits monosomy while the other one exhibits trisomy. (**Hint:** A sperm will fertilize the "egg" and add its chromosome in the last step.)*

Nondisjunction